MAPPING THE

BRAIN

AND ITS FUNCTIONS

INTEGRATING ENABLING TECHNOLOGIES INTO NEUROSCIENCE RESEARCH

Constance M. Pechura and Joseph B. Martin, Editors

Committee on a National Neural Circuitry Database
Division of Health Sciences Policy
Division of Biobehavioral Sciences and Mental Disorders

INSTITUTE OF MEDICINE

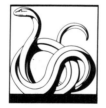

NATIONAL ACADEMY PRESS
Washington, D.C.   1991

NATIONAL ACADEMY PRESS • 2101 Constitution Avenue, N.W. • Washington, DC 20418

NOTICE: The project that is the subject of this report was approved by the Governing Board of the National Research Council, whose members are drawn from the councils of the National Academy of Sciences, the National Academy of Engineering, and the Institute of Medicine. The members of the committee responsible for the report were chosen for their special competences and with regard for appropriate balance.

This report has been reviewed by a group other than the authors according to procedures approved by a Report Review Committee consisting of members of the National Academy of Sciences, the National Academy of Engineering, and the Institute of Medicine.

The Institute of Medicine was chartered in 1970 by the National Academy of Sciences to enlist distinguished members of the appropriate professions in the examination of policy matters pertaining to the health of the public. In this, the Institute acts under both the Academy's 1863 congressional charter responsibility to be an advisor to the federal government and its own initiative in identifying issues of medical care, research, and education.

The work on which this publication is based was performed pursuant to Contract No. 278-89-003 with the National Institute of Mental Health, Public Health Service, Department of Health and Human Services. Funds for this contract were provided by the National Institute of Mental Health, the National Institute of Drug Abuse, and the National Science Foundation (under NSF Agreement No. BNS-8913554).

Library of Congress Cataloging-in-Publication Data
Institute of Medicine (U.S.). Committee on a National Neural
  Circuitry Database.
    Mapping the brain and its functions: integrating enabling
  technologies into neuroscience research / Committee on a National
  Neural Circuitry Database, Division of Health Sciences Policy,
  Division of Biobehavioral Sciences and Mental Health, Institute of
  Medicine; Constance M. Pechura and Joseph D. Martin, editors.
        p.   cm. — (Publication ; no. IOM-91-08)
    Includes bibliographical references and index.
    ISBN 0-309-04497-9
    1. Brain—Research—Data processing—Congresses. 2. Brain
  mapping—Congresses. I. Pechura, Constance M. II. Martin, Joseph
  B., 1938- . III. Title. IV. Series: IOM publication ; 91-08.
    [DNLM: 1. Brain—physiology. 2. Brain Mapping. 3. Medical
  Informatics. 4. Neurosciences. 5. Research. WL 335 I59m]
  QP376.I516   1991
  612.8'2—dc20
  DNLM/DLC
  for Library of Congress   91-4832
                                                            CIP

Printed in the United States of America

The serpent has been a symbol of long life, healing, and knowledge among almost all cultures and religions since the beginning of recorded history. The image adopted as a logotype by the Institute of Medicine is based on a relief carving from ancient Greece, now held by the Staatlichemuseen in Berlin.

Committee on a National Neural Circuitry Database

Institute of Medicine Staff

Ruth Ellen Bulger, Director, Division of Health Sciences Policy
Constance M. Pechura, Study Director
Charles E. Vela, Staff Officer[‡]
Elizabeth E. Meyer, Research Associate
Shelley A. Myers, Project Assistant
April E. Powers, Project Assistant

---

[*]Member, Institute of Medicine.
[†]Member, Institute of Medicine and National Academy of Sciences.
[‡]From September 1989 to May 1990.

Preface

The Committee on a National Neural Circuitry Database was convened in October 1989 to formulate a position concerning the feasibility and utility of incorporating computer technology into the basic and clinical neurosciences in order to enhance research progress. The committee was comprised of experts from the fields of neuroscience and computer and information sciences. Each group was, in general, unaccustomed to the other area of endeavor, and considerable effort was required in the beginning to identify the problems confronting neuroscience and to learn more about the electronic and digital applications that might be relevant. To carry the analysis forward, the committee commissioned four task forces to examine the issues in more detail, organized three symposia and open hearings, and sought advice and counsel from leaders of the neuroscience community and from those with experience in database development and computer systems design. This report summarizes the committee's findings and offers advice regarding the opportunity to facilitate neuroscience research and to maximize the benefits of that research.

It was not altogether clear at the outset of the study how the recommendations would unfold. Several members of the committee were skeptical that the time was ripe to apply new technologies to the gathering and dissemination of neuroscience data. The enthusiasm that emerges in the report for new approaches to these issues arose from much deliberation, numerous discussions, and careful assessment of the technological opportunities that currently exist and which are expected to expand rapidly in the future. Throughout the study the committee confronted some of the same challenges that will eventually be faced by those who may be charged with implementing its recommendations. One challenge was to find effective means of communication across the diverse disciplines of neuroscience (basic and clinical) and computer science and informatics (encompassing digital graphics, database technology, and electronic networks). Beyond the expected difficulties of language (i.e., certain words mean one thing to neuroscientists and something entirely different to computer scientists), there were often fundamental differences in the perceptual frameworks used by the two groups. In educating each other the members of the committee came to the end of the study with a much greater understanding of how each discipline approaches its work and how these approaches can and should be melded in a common effort.

A second challenge was to balance creativity with practicality in order to forge a reasonable plan for application of electronic and digital technologies to the neurosciences. Such a balance had to be achieved largely in the absence of immediately applicable models from other areas of biomedical science. The committee evaluated the existing biomedical databases and found substantial disparity in their development, funding, and structures. This disparity was particularly characteristic of the genome and protein sequence databases. The committee also discovered that the federal infrastructure for support of biomedical science has not yet developed a clear, integrated set of guidelines and policies to facilitate the incorporation of technological advances. Nevertheless, technology has made major inroads in most of the physical and biological sciences.

A third challenge the committee faced was the recognition that its deliberations were being held during a time of serious biomedical research funding constraints. Indeed, the question of funding was at the core of the most vigorous objections to the proposed brain mapping initiative: some neuroscientists feared the initiative would produce large-scale efforts that would undermine the traditional investigator-initiated research enterprise. The committee took these concerns seriously and the prospect of allocating already scarce resources to possible new initiatives led the committee to attempt to assess the probable costs and benefits of its recommendations. In addressing this issue there emerged a recurring theme of the advantages of investment now, as a protection against costly corrections later. The recommendations offered in the report reflect the committee's attention to the possible dangers, as well as the possible benefits that neuroscience can derive from computer and information technology.

Notwithstanding the difficulties presented by these challenges, great enthusiasm emerged from the committee's deliberations. The committee believes that the more than 150 neuroscientists who served on the committee, participated in task force groups, attended open hearings, or responded to written solicitations of opinions were representative of the diverse neuroscience community. Some were already in favor of the proposals being discussed and expressed strong views that the proposals should proceed. This group tended to be comprised of the most experienced in the use of computer and information technology. Some participants had strong reservations about the proposals. Of the remaining participants, many held no clear position in the beginning. In the end, however, some of the greatest excitement could be found among this group as they considered the capabilities of the various technologies shown in demonstrations and presentations and how these capabilities could be applied to data collection and analysis, as well as to rapid communication of research results.

The recommendations that resulted from the committee's deliberations and activities address certain key issues. The first is that a proper base of hands-on experience must be built before any large-scale effort can begin. Thus, the committee has proposed a two-phase initiative. Phase 1 would consist of pilot projects that would allow neuroscientists and computer scientists to work together to construct usable resource prototypes and address a variety of technological and sociological challenges as described in the report. To realize the greatest benefit from these pilot projects, however, a strong central coordinating body must be in place. Thus, the committee has recommended that an advisory panel be charged with certain responsibilities, including the facilitation of information exchange among the projects, the establishment of editorial and training functions, the development of policies to protect confidentiality and intellectual property, and the definition of the overall direction of the program. The committee's recommendations further outline the possible funding structures that might be used and the need for additional appropriations to support the proposed projects.

Despite the need for program stability and central authority, the committee did not assign responsibility for the proposed initiative to any single agency or institute but instead outlined two possible structures. In one, a lead agency would have authority over the implementation of the initiative and responsibility for its funding. Alternatively, multiple agencies could share funding responsibility, but central authority would be maintained by formal agreements between two or more agencies or institutes. Because neuroscience research is funded through a wide variety of sources, the committee felt that strict definition of a structure might limit resources available to the proposed initiatives. Similarly, a detailed plan for the second phase of the initiative is not offered in the committee's recommendations. The more global second phase of development and integration of electronic and digital resources must proceed from the experience gained in the pilot projects, a requirement which limited the committee's ability to define a precise structure for the future.

The increasing use of many of the technologies discussed in this report is beginning to change the way research is conducted and an integral role for such technologies in biomedical science in general, and neuroscience in particular, is inevitable. In the absence of clear priorities and policies to support these technologies, the process of change will occur in a scattered, disparate, and costly manner. It is the committee's hope that this report will underscore the importance of a new focus on the role of computer and information technology in the conduct of neuroscience research. Such a focus would help bring neuroscience to an unprecedented level of discovery and, in a broader sense, provide a model for technological integration that would benefit all of biomedical science.

In that spirit, this report is aimed primarily toward policymakers in the Congress, the Public Health Service, and other federal agencies who are responsible for the support and direction of the biomedical research enterprise. The report will also be of interest to basic and clinical neuroscientists, computer scientists, systems developers, and information scientists. Beyond these groups, other individuals interested in the broad issues of technological change may find certain aspects of the report useful. Therefore, the committee attempted to respond to the needs of a wide audience in constructing this report. Chapters 1 and 2 emphasize certain key aspects of neuroscience research, including already achieved and potential benefits; the chapters further describe how computer and information technology might enhance the acquisition of more information about the brain than is available today. Chapter 3 is an overview of some of the methods and concepts of neuroscience. This chapter is specifically intended to give those readers not familiar with neuroscience a greater appreciation of the field's complexity, a factor that makes the integration of computer and information technology especially challenging. Chapter 4 provides a fictional scenario of how a laboratory of the future might use electronic and digital resources, followed by descriptions and specific examples of how computer and information technologies are now in greater use in biomedical science. A summary of the input received by the committee through its various activities is contained in Chapter 5. This chapter covers a broad range of topics that were discussed at task force meetings and open hearings and that provided a strong base of knowledge for crafting specific recommendations. Finally, Chapter 6 contains the committee's formal recommendations.

In completing this study, the committee was aided in many valuable ways. Of particular benefit were the efforts of the task force participants (see Appendix A). These neuroscientists, computer scientists, and information scientists gave generously of their time and expertise to provide the committee with creative and in many cases indispensable suggestions. Another important source of input was those individuals in the neuroscience community who responded to the committee's requests for opinions. These responses kept the committee in touch with the variety of viewpoints existing in the field. The committee also appreciated the help given by the speakers and demonstrators at each of the three symposia and open hearings (see Appendix C), as well as the insightful, honest input provided by all the participants of these meetings. Finally, the committee wishes to thank the Fidia Pharmaceutical Corporation and the Fidia Research Foundation for their support of the symposia and hearings, and Barry Peterson and Sandra Hicks from the Department of Physiology at Northwestern University for their help in arranging the hearing held in Chicago.

During the course of the study, other individuals provided helpful information and necessary background materials. These included Stephen Koslow and Ronald Schoenfeld, the study's project officers from the National Institute of Mental Health; Lana Skirboll from the Alcohol, Drug Abuse, and Mental Health Administration; Lawrence Sellin from the National Science Foundation; Daniel Masys from the National Library of Medicine; Eugene Streicher from the National Institute of Neurological Disorders and Stroke; and Bruce Waxman from the Defense Mapping Agency. The committee is also grateful for the work of the seven individuals who reviewed the report and provided many thoughtful, carefully crafted suggestions and commentaries, which greatly strengthened the final product.

The committee's charge could not have been met without the dedication and expertise of the staff of the Institute of Medicine. Special thanks are owed to staff editor Leah Mazade for her careful work in polishing the report. The committee also wishes to thank the director of the Division of Health Sciences Policy, Ruth Bulger, for her consistent interest and excellent suggestions. Shelley Myers, the project assistant, made the many meetings in and out of Washington as comfortable for the participants as possible and provided excellent secretarial support. April Powers became the project assistant toward the end of the study, when a thousand details, in ever-changing report drafts, require attention. She dealt with these pressures with singular commitment and a calming sense of humor. The numerous contributions made by Elizabeth Meyer, the study's research associate, would be difficult to list here. To each task she was assigned, from planning figures and illustrations to writing summaries of the many meetings and designing the fliers for open hearings, Elizabeth brought a quiet competence and an unfailing willingness to help. Before leaving the study to accept a position in industry, Charles Vela, staff officer and assistant study director, provided valuable assistance as a liaison to the computer and information scientists of the committee and key information regarding the funding and organization of other scientific databases. Lastly, and most importantly, I wish to acknowledge the extraordinary efforts of Constance Pechura, the study director, in shepherding the committee through its difficult task.

Joseph B. Martin, *Chairman*
Committee on
National Neural Circuitry Database

Contents

List of Boxes, Color Plates, Figures, and Tables

MAPPING THE
BRAIN
AND ITS FUNCTIONS

Summary

The human brain is a fascinating, complex system whose mysteries are becoming increasingly accessible to the tools of modern science. Neuroscientists have amassed a sizable body of knowledge about the structure of the brain and its specific functions, which has improved our ability to treat a variety of mental and neurological diseases. Many other diseases are less tractable, however, and effective treatments will require major advances in both basic and clinical neuroscience. Underlying these advances will be an explosion of experimental data, whose magnitude poses serious problems for information management and communication.

Effective access to existing neuroscience information is critical to the enterprise of discovery: such information forms the basis of new hypotheses, drives the search for improved methodologies, and, ultimately, leads to insights applicable to human disease. New strategies must be developed to enhance integration of this information and to facilitate new discoveries about the brain. Within the range of potentially beneficial strategies, the greater use of computer and information technology in neuroscience research holds particular promise.

This report synthesizes the deliberations of the Institute of Medicine's Committee on a National Neural Circuitry Database, which was formed at the request of the National Institute of Mental Health (NIMH), the National Institute on Drug Abuse (NIDA), and the National Science Foundation (NSF). The committee's task was to consider the desirability, feasibility, and possible ways of implementing a family of resources, both electronic (e.g., computer networks) and digital (e.g., databases),

1

for the enhancement of neuroscience research. The incorporation of computer and information technology into diverse scientific fields is often accomplished in the absence of coordinated policy through trial and error by individual scientists capitalizing on rapidly developing technological innovation. These efforts have often led to far-reaching changes in the style of scientific research that call for new governmental policies regarding the conduct of research in this country and abroad. Within this context, and with an overall purpose of increasing the resources available to the neuroscience community, this committee has sought to

- formulate a position on the requirements for and appropriateness of establishing a family of electronic and digital resources for basic and clinical neuroscience that would allow optimal data communication and sharing among investigators;
- consider the scope and elements of data that would constitute these resources and determine strategies for representing the diverse data types generated by neuroscientists;
- consider data storage, retrieval, and sharing schemes of existing national databases to identify successful strategies and potential pitfalls for the possible establishment of computerized resources for neuroscience;
- describe the optimal organization of a family of computerized resources so that it can be efficiently established and coordinated for research use by the neuroscience research community, clinical investigators, clinicians, students, and educators; and
- provide recommendations to NIMH, NIDA, and NSF on future directions in program development with respect to establishing such electronic and digital resources.

Advancing Neuroscience in the Decade of the Brain

The major advances in neuroscience in the past two decades have generated the opportunity that now exists to achieve an integrated understanding of the brain's structure and functions. These advances, which are producing new data on brain activity, include

- the identification of complex anatomical connections;
- capabilities for understanding the biochemical, molecular, and genetic mechanisms that control brain structure and functions;
- the ability to measure and visualize human brain functioning during mental activity; and
- the ability to monitor neural activity simultaneously in complicated networks of neurons.

These and other advances have occurred primarily through the efforts of individual investigators working in small groups on highly specific projects. Despite the piecemeal quality of these efforts, the information derived from them is so extensive that it is extremely difficult to coordinate it all and produce a meaningful picture of how the brain functions. This traditional method of neuroscience research— individual investigators, highly specific projects—is similar to a group of surveyors, each of whom has been assigned to chart a different geographical region. To chart an entire continent, however, the work of each surveyor must somehow be coordinated with the work of all other surveyors. Based on input obtained through a variety of means, as well as on its own deliberations, the committee considers it necessary to establish a formal Brain Mapping Initiative to coordinate the valuable efforts of individual neuroscientists in such a way that new discoveries occur with greater speed and efficiency. The Brain Mapping Initiative is meant to subsume all the proposed aspects of a National Neural Circuitry Database. In addition, it expresses explicitly the overarching goals of the proposed effort and reflects more adequately the complex of electronic and digital resources that will be required.

Complexity drives the need for information management

The brain is more complicated than any other part of the human body. To understand the brain, scientists must measure and analyze the rapid changes in neuronal activity that occur throughout the brain's many intricate neural networks and pathways. The scope of such an endeavor is daunting. Neuroscience research proceeds along a multi-level hierarchy, from behavior and emotion to molecular interactions and genetic expression. At each level, researchers use numerous techniques that are specifically designed to collect information appropriate to that level. But information from one level may, and most often does, have important implications for research and knowledge at other levels. Therefore, new methods for assembling and integrating the pieces of the "brain puzzle" can be as important as the individual discoveries themselves.

The goal of information management, which is distinct from simply acquiring data, is to realize the greatest possible benefit from the data that already exist. The field of neuroscience research has two major information management needs: (1) databases, which relate diverse data types systematically and efficiently, and (2) visualization of structures in three dimensions to capture the discoverable architecture of the brain and relate this architecture to brain functioning.

Examples of the Value of Integrating Knowledge to Solve Problems

It is useful to examine how the diverse neural hierarchy relates to real biological processes and human disease. The examples in this section provide a glimpse of the breadth of neuroscience research and suggest how that research, coupled with better information management, can have positive effects on human health.

Vision: How we see affects how we think

Interpretation, complex perception, and even the appreciation of beauty often begins with visual information. The neural basis of vision involves billions of neurons and more than 300 separate but interrelated pathways in the cerebral cortex alone. As in all neural systems, visual functioning relies on the coordinated activity of neurons that communicate with each other, employing hundreds of different molecules for the generation of specific electrical and chemical signals. Many of these molecules are arranged in distinctive patterns and located in specific brain regions. The combination of complex physiological processes, anatomical pathways, and molecular and chemical interactions creates a system that functions extremely well but that is exceedingly difficult to decipher. Notwithstanding all of the information currently available, the fundamental nature of visual perception remains a mystery. To understand it, we need more experimental data and new ways of assembling the diverse kinds of related data into an integrated whole.

Among the resources necessary to understand the basis of pattern recognition and to gain insight into existing control and regulatory mechanisms are methods for overlaying anatomical maps with chemical and physiological maps. Computer simulations would also be of great value for understanding the signal processing of neural sets and networks. (Such simulations could also be used outside of neuroscience to construct new kinds of sensors and signal processors for robots and other automated devices.) Enhancing research into vision with these electronic tools promises to help ameliorate visual deficits caused by injury and to increase the range of treatments available for a number of diseases, including glaucoma, diabetic retinopathy, and inherited retinal degeneration, as well as blindness from other causes.

Substance abuse: The search for the biology of self-destruction

A large fraction of the U.S. population uses substances that are injurious to health. These substances include legally approved drugs, such as nicotine and alcohol, and illegal drugs, such as cocaine and heroin, that are accompanied by the societal burdens of violent crime and increased infant mortality, among others. The key to substance abuse lies in the brain. One of the clear successes of neuroscience has been the discovery that certain molecules on the surface of neurons, called receptors, specifically bind many drugs, including nicotine, heroin and other opiates, and even benzodiazepines, such as Valium®. This finding has led to the search for synthetic compounds that can block the actions of an injurious drug, yet still satisfy a person's craving for that drug. Neuroscientists have also begun to pay close attention to those areas of the brain that mediate not only the normal pleasurable experiences of eating and socialization but the motivating, often pleasurable, drug effects that can lead to psychological addiction. The complexity of these brain areas, however, greatly complicates the investigations.

Unlike the visual and motor systems of the brain, the so-called reward system of brain nuclei and cortical areas has not been clearly defined. Two kinds of computerized databases could help researchers construct a framework for this system. One would depict the distribution patterns of important receptors and compare these patterns to the known anatomical and neurochemical circuitry of the brain. The other would contain information specific to those areas of the brain known to be involved in addictive processes. These resources would allow investigators faced with integrating data on anatomy, neurochemistry, pharmacology, and behavior to benefit from the research of other subspecialties in the field.

Pain: Sometimes a warning, sometimes a curse

Pain is a ubiquitous reality of life, and we need it to a certain degree to recognize sprained ankles, overstressed back muscles, kidney stones, infections, and many other problems. Yet for tens of thousands of people who suffer from abnormal or pathological pain, any benefit from pain is hard to identify. For these individuals, pain is an intractable barrier to a happy, productive life. The neural basis of pain involves almost every region of the brain, spinal cord, and peripheral nerves. Often, pain affects other body systems, such as the immune and endocrine systems. The complexity of pain perception helps to explain the variety in the pain people experience and the treatments that have been developed. Much has been learned in recent years about the basic neural mechanisms of pain, but substantial gaps in knowledge remain. For example, we still do not understand pathological pain—the severe pain often experienced in an amputated body part (despite its absence, so-called phantom limb pain) or the terrible pain that can occur following seemingly minor injuries or after surgical procedures.

There is a pressing need to transfer the information gained through basic research about pain to clinical practice. At present, widely divergent strategies are used to treat pain and to use it diagnostically. A broad range of professionals are often involved; thus, the responsibility for pain management may shift as a patient is moved from the operating room, to recovery, to a postsurgery ward. A database that related clinical observations to an integrated picture of relevant basic scientific data would be of great value in pain management, especially if it were combined with a repository of treatment and diagnostic strategies and their documented outcomes. Indeed, better ways to integrate data from basic pain research could contribute significantly to the alleviation of a major cause of human suffering.

Schizophrenia: Broken minds, shattered dreams

The symptoms of schizophrenia often emerge in adolescence or early adulthood, just as young people are beginning to plan their futures. In this country the lives of more than 2 million people have been devastated by schizophrenia and its various manifestations, which include hallucinations, delusions, blunted emotions, cognitive deficits, and an inability to maintain meaningful relationships. Neuroscience has focused on three major research areas in its search for understanding: neurochemical abnormalities, structural and functional brain abnormalities, and potential genetic and environmental causes.

It has long been thought that the effects of the neurotransmitter dopamine are greater than normal in the brains of those with schizophrenia. Not all of the symptoms of schizophrenia are alleviated by depression of dopamine activity, however, and evidence is mounting that other neurotransmitters are involved. The structural abnormalities identified thus far in some individuals are enlarged cerebral ventricles and a thinning of the cerebral cortex in certain areas. Although there seems to be a concomitant decrease in functioning in the frontal cortex, neuroscientists do not know how these structural and functional abnormalities contribute to the causes or symptoms of schizophrenia.

Advances such as gene mapping and positron emission tomography (PET) scanning may lead to increased understanding of the neurobiology of schizophrenia, but greater integration of the available information is needed. The kinds of digital resources that would be of most use are maps of the distribution of dopamine, dopamine receptors, and other neuroregulators in the brain, databases of the existing brain imaging data with detailed descriptions of each patient's history and specific constellation of symptoms, and databases containing information about the genes that are most likely to confer susceptibility to schizophrenia. For those whose ravaged lives testify to the burden of this disease, and for their families, needed answers are long overdue.

The Growth of Neuroscience

Neuroscience research has grown in response to critical problems

The preceding examples reflect only a small portion of the overall cost of mental and neurological diseases. These diseases, combined with drug abuse, constitute an immense financial burden to our population every year in direct care expenses and lost wages. Nearly 23 million Americans suffer from head and spinal cord injuries, hearing and speech disorders, or infectious diseases of the nervous system. More than 3.5 million people suffer from Alzheimer's, Huntington's, or Parkinson's disease, or from other degenerative disorders, including multiple sclerosis and amyotrophic lateral sclerosis. More than 60 million people suffer from mental illnesses, including schizophrenia and depression, and more than 20 million abuse alcohol or drugs. Each of these problems clamors for resolution.

In response, neuroscience has made steady progress in a number of areas. Researchers have applied many new technologies, from the first oscilloscope to modern computer graphics, to the study of the brain. These technologies, combined with insightful, painstaking research, have led to the important breakthroughs witnessed in the past two or three decades and have enlarged considerably our understanding of the biological basis of disease. In addition, many talented young scientists have entered the field of neuroscience: the membership of the Society for Neuroscience has risen from 500 in 1969 to more than 17,500 in 1990. Because we now possess vast amounts of data and thousands of bright, dedicated scientists, the opportunities for successfully addressing the remaining questions about the brain have never been more promising.

Neuroscience is a national priority

Another source of the existing opportunities in neuroscience is the high priority the United States places on research aimed at alleviating mental and neurological disorders. Research support has come from various government bodies, including the National Institutes of

Health (NIH), the Alcohol, Drug Abuse, and Mental Health Administration (ADAMHA), the Department of Veterans Affairs, the National
Science Foundation, and other government agencies; private agencies
and foundations, including the Howard Hughes Medical Institute,
the MacArthur Foundation, and the Pew Charitable Trusts, have also
provided funds. It is estimated that these groups invest more than
$1.5 billion annually in neuroscience research, the majority of which
comes from NIH and ADAMHA. Yet however impressive the total,
this investment represents a very small fraction of the overall societal
costs of neurological and mental diseases. In times of competing
needs and fiscal constraints, it is important to find ways to derive the
most value from the investments that are made. The committee believes that a Brain Mapping Initiative, by enhancing the process of
discovery and the communication of new insights in neuroscience,
can help to maximize the benefits gained from the present investment
of national resources.

Computer and Information Technology
in Biomedical and Neuroscience Research

In the committee's opinion, a complex of electronic resources that
will enhance neuroscience research is an attainable goal. Current
trends in computer and information sciences clearly point to an unprecedented opportunity to incorporate technologies that will enable
neuroscientists to expand their use of valuable, hard-won data and to
communicate these data more effectively to other scientists. In addition, the sheer mass of neuroscience information accumulated to date,
and the accelerating rate at which new results are being obtained and
reported, are becoming major driving forces for the kind of organization, structure, and accessibility that electronic and digital resources
can provide. Increasing sophistication in computer technology, coupled
with decreasing costs, holds out the promise of enhanced research
capabilities for many fields of scientific endeavor—but in particular,
for neuroscience, owing to its inherently visual, hierarchical nature.

Three areas of computer science are especially important for biomedical research: computer graphics, database technology, and electronic
networking. The use of computer graphics, so pervasive in such
fields as earth mapping and space sciences, has only recently emerged
as a resource in biomedical research, a direct result of the rapidly
decreasing costs of computer memory capacities. One of the most
successful applications of computer graphics has been the modeling
of molecular structures using data derived from x-ray crystallography. No longer are scientists confined to trying to visualize a dyna-

mic molecule from a ball-and-stick depiction; computer models can be rotated and manipulated to simulate the molecule's actual functioning. These models will soon help to predict which drugs stop certain viruses, how genes are turned on and off, and how two molecules may interact with one another. In neuroscience, the use of computer graphics has led to visualization of the activity of the human brain through PET scanning and magnetic resonance imaging (MRI). Such graphic depictions have proved to be so useful that greater and greater attention is being paid to the concept of visualization computing in biomedical sciences. One example of this increased attention is the greater priority given to biomedical computing by leading universities and government laboratories.

Databases, the second computer science area that is important to biomedical research, allow digitized data to be stored and organized in a way that makes the data easily accessible. Databases can be word, number, image, or sound oriented, and can be either public or private. The use of databases, including databases of biomedical information, has increased substantially over the past 15 years. The leader in the development of biomedical databases has been the National Library of Medicine (NLM), which currently maintains a number of on-line systems, including bibliographic databases of scientific literature, registries of chemicals and their toxic effects, and medical information related to cancer and other diseases. Other prominent scientific databases are the protein sequence and genome databases developed by a variety of institutions and individuals, which are being used in the efforts to map the human genome. The need for databases for neuroscience information is great, and the systems are beginning to emerge. Neuroscience database developers can learn much from the experiences of the NLM and protein and genome database originators.

The purpose of computer networks is to help create a communication environment that is as free of barriers as possible. In science the communication of data and ideas is as important to the growth of knowledge as the data themselves; consequently, the use of computer networks holds great promise for neuroscience. Since 1969, networks connecting research laboratories and universities have grown so rapidly that today more than 5,000 interconnected networks in 35 countries connect more than 300,000 computers. Further efforts, such as the National Research and Education Network (NREN), are under way to upgrade the transmission rates of U.S. scientific and educational computer networks, including the National Science Foundation's NSFNET, to permit them to handle more data and data of greater complexity (e.g., image data, which currently cannot be efficiently transmitted through computer networks). If computer networks are to be a viable method for communication of neuroscience data, the planned increase in transmission rates is a necessity. Also needed are strategies for standard data formats to facilitate communication of digitized information among investigators.

Building Consensus, Identifying Needs

The committee sponsored a number of consultative activities to seek out the opinions and advice of the neuroscience community at large. These activities included written requests for opinions (published in various journals and solicited directly from the leadership of the Society for Neuroscience); formation of four task forces; and sponsorship of three symposia and open hearings, which were held in Washington, D.C., Chicago, and San Francisco. In addition, the committee commissioned two background papers: one traced the development and current uses of genome and related scientific databases, and the other investigated the Defense Mapping Agency's experience in converting cartographic data to digital formats. Participants in these activities reflected a wide range of backgrounds and expertise including library management, scientific database administration and design, computer science, and neuroscience research. Additionally, participants came from academic departments, government laboratories, and private industry.

The complexity of neuroscience dictates that the scope of data included in any group of electronic and digital resources must eventually be quite broad. The majority of the individuals providing input to the committee's deliberations envisioned the proposed complex of resources as necessarily containing more kinds of information than are already or can be contained in library reference materials and published journals. Participants also endorsed using the neuroanatomy of the brain as the principal organizing arrangement for the resources. Information on neuroanatomy could function as the skeleton or frame-work on which data from multiple levels of the brain's hierarchy, including information on functions, could be displayed. The information would include neural pathways, cell types, neurochemistry and identification of neurotransmitters, protein and gene sequences and gene mapping, receptor types, electrophysiological responses, and data regarding behavioral relationships, such as memory.

To realize such a database, the computerized resources must include a range of capabilities. Some of the features participants deemed necessary were the ability to

- transform data into three-dimensional images,

- browse through various kinds of data,
- extract arbitrarily defined subsets of data, and
- compare different brain images with each other by precise overlaying or co-registration of the images.

There was overwhelming consensus among all participants that a single National Neural Circuitry Database was not a workable plan. Rather, a complex of electronic and digital resources should be developed to include separate databases with varied levels of accessibility. This complex should be composed of reference databases, data banks, informal databases, national and international registries, research collaboration databases, and specialty databases.

To implement this complex of resources, however, significant advances will be required. The committee identified three areas deserving of attention: databases, networks, and imaging technologies. Only imaging is sufficiently advanced to be immediately applied to neuroscience research. Database management technology presents one of the most difficult barriers to implementation. Currently available database technology cannot handle images easily, although improved capabilities are under development. Database developers should consider incorporating these advances as soon as they become available. In addition, present mechanisms to interlink different databases will need to be improved substantially for application to neuroscience. Human–computer interfaces also require improvement so that they are uncomplicated for users yet powerful enough to enable the user to extract needed information. Underlying both database and user interface design issues is the challenge of developing software that allows the data to be accessible and usable. Finally, as noted earlier, computer network upgrading will be necessary for the transmission of complex image data.

The final technical topic covered by the task forces was the development of standards for the exchange of data. Four areas of technical concern were addressed:

- Data representation and standard data formats are needed for textual and numerical data and for the generation of images and graphics.
- Mechanisms are needed for conveying new algorithms for a variety of applications.
- Standard human–computer interface packages should be explored to reduce barriers to the actual use of electronic resources.
- Standard communication protocols are needed to accommodate the dynamic range of data accessibility required for research-oriented databases.

In addition to the technological changes that will be required to implement the proposed resources, the task forces identified sociological patterns and issues specific to the scientific community that must also be addressed. The development of standard data formats presents important sociological questions. Participants expressed strong views that standards should evolve out of the needs and perspectives of users and not be imposed from outside. A careful balance must be sought between the need for technical standards to facilitate communication and the barriers that can result from overly strict standard formats.

Data sharing is another major sociological issue. In some neuroscience specialties, sharing of unpublished and "raw" data is commonplace, whereas in other specialties such openness is rare. Although the committee places no value judgment on either end of the data-sharing continuum—restrictive to open—it recognizes the existence of a continuum and concludes that potential data-sharing mechanisms must be carefully considered as part of any initiative. For example, priority should be given to formulating methods to ensure that proper credit is assigned for those contributing data and that the privacy of human subjects is protected. In addition, the level of certification (peer-reviewed, verified, unverified, etc.) of all data must be clearly stated, although preliminary data probably would be included in special databases. Clear identification of different levels of certainty, including unambiguous labeling of preliminary data, will also need to be incorporated into the various kinds of databases; for major resources, editorial boards may be a good mechanism to aid in this process. As in all sciences, replication of experimental results will continue to be important. The task forces also supported the concept that university tenure committees should consider certain types of data sharing, particularly of peer-reviewed data, as evidence of professional competence, comparable to journal publication and teaching evaluations. The committee was further encouraged to examine the policies developed recently by some journals devoted to gene mapping and gene and protein sequencing for deposit of data into established databases. Other areas of sociological concern were how to ensure that electronic resources would be accessible to more than a few well-funded laboratories and how to overcome resistance to the integration of technology into the way people work. An additional concern of many participants was the changing work force that would result from greater use of technology and the need for computer specialists with expertise in neurobiology as well as neurobiologists with expertise in computer science.

To overcome these technological and sociological impediments, the task forces in particular strongly recommended that the committee call for the establishment of pilot projects. The primary goal of these projects would be to provide a desperately needed base of experience from which to establish a family of usable computerized resources. The task forces suggested a two-phase effort, with the pilot projects as a necessary first step, followed by a more global incorporation of computerized resources into the neuroscience research enterprise.

A key area of consensus was that pilot projects would require coordination and that oversight and evaluation mechanisms were crucial to the eventual implementation of the resource complex. Structures suggested for coordination of the pilot projects included advisory boards, host institutions, and formal meetings.

A final area of discussion was funding. Despite general support for the proposed effort, many participants expressed concern about how and where funds might be secured. There was considerable dialogue about current constraints on biomedical research support, and virtually all participants expressed the opinion that funds for this project should be obtained only through additional appropriations.

The Brain Mapping Initiative: Committee Recommendations

After considering the opinions expressed and the input received through its activities and during its own deliberations, the committee concluded that an environment of opportunity now exists to enhance neuroscience research by a more global incorporation of computer and information technologies. Considering past experiences in other scientific disciplines, however, it is also apparent that to ensure the greatest benefit from these technologies, they should be incorporated with care and with a clear vision of the intended goal. Neuroscience is diverse in its methodology and levels of inquiry. To achieve true understanding, all of the available information must be coordinated into an integrated, meaningful picture. At present, the detailed information being generated at every level of neural organization is difficult to grasp and integrate. Even searches for information regarding relatively specific neural levels or processes are hindered because the information is widely scattered through scores of different journals, review papers, symposia summaries, and books. Added to these difficulties are the unique visual requirements of neuroscience. The mass of information is steadily expanding because researchers can now generate two- and three-dimensional graphic images relatively quickly and easily. The increasing use of computers to collect the various kinds of neuroscience data needed by researchers and the development currently under way of the technology to link these computerized research environments makes this an opportune time to begin a Brain Mapping Initiative. Therefore,

> **the committee recommends that the Brain Mapping Initiative be established with the long-term objective of developing three-dimensional computerized maps and models of the structure, functions, connectivity, pharmacology, and molecular biology of human, rat, and monkey[1] brains across developmental stages and reflecting both normal and disease states.**

The Brain Mapping Initiative is meant to include features that were originally proposed for a National Neural Circuitry Database, although the new initiative, unlike the earlier project, would not be a single-entity database. Rather, the Brain Mapping Initiative would lead to the establishment of a complex of interrelated, integrated databases accessible from individual laboratories. The committee is aware of the broad scale of such an undertaking and that the successful implementation of this program will require transformation of the way information is acquired, communicated, and analyzed by neuroscientists. Therefore, the committee envisions the initiative as a long-term endeavor to be accomplished in two phases. Phase 1 would comprise an organized initiation of seed or pilot projects with the overall goals of gaining experience in the incorporation of the required technologies and applying that experience to long-range planning for phase 2. Phase 2 would involve construction of the maps and models necessary to provide a complex of digital and electronic resources to enhance neuroscience research. To begin phase 1,

> **the committee recommends the establishment of pilot projects or consortia. These projects should be peer-reviewed by neuroscientists and computer scientists; they should also be investigator initiated, involve geographically dispersed laboratories, and include neuroscientists with varied levels of computer experience. The projects should develop common formats for the exchange of data and focus on different types of computer data representations (geometric, structural, image, and free text). Selection of projects should be on the basis of research quality and value to the evolution of a complex of electronic resources for mapping the brain.**

The pilot projects the committee recommends should be a coordinated program of separate efforts but with certain common goals. In the committee's vision, the pilot program would consist of several groups of investigators, each working on specific neuroscience topics, with the primary goals of mapping the brain's anatomy, chemistry, and functions, and forging pathways for the integration of computer and information technology into the overall neuroscience research effort. Consortia could be organized among geographically distinct institutions or as centers housed within a single institution. (If the centers approach is chosen, special attention should be given to involving investigators from geographically distant institutions as users of the technologies developed.) Research topics for the phase 1 projects should reflect the vertical hierarchy of the brain from behavior and emotion to molecular biological and genetic mechanisms, as well as the horizontal range of inquiry including the anatomy, physiology, neurochemistry, and molecular and developmental biology of specific brain systems.

In terms of technical developments, the overall goals of the pilot project program would be the following:

• Develop electronic data collection and storage methods for data types at each level of the neural hierarchy.

• Identify the kinds of data, level of resolution, and experimental information necessary to facilitate new insights and stimulate research.

• Examine and evaluate the wide range of available capabilities that can increase use of the resources and enhance access to meaningful information.

• Develop a variety of databases from formal, consensus databases to informal databases for research collaboration.

• Develop and experiment with different software for translation across different computing environments, for user interfaces, for network transmission of images, for data searching, and for image generation and comparison.

• Begin to develop standard data formats, nomenclature, and data collection schemes, and to evaluate the evolution of these standards.

• Gain experience in data sharing and communication through electronic means, including networks and transportable media.

• Communicate with others in the program to share and evaluate experiences and technological developments.

To ensure the greatest benefits possible from the phase 1 projects, the committee agreed to emphasize certain areas by formulating the recommendations below.

The committee recognizes that neuroscience efforts proceed internationally and recommends that an international registry of neuroscience databases and contacts be established so that appropriate linkages can be created in the future.

Such a registry, which should be available to users through computer networks, would help to identify currently available resources and provide a mechanism to coordinate the efforts of phase 1 investigators and investigators in other countries.

The committee recommends the establishment of an archive of public domain software, accessible through computer networks.

The committee expects that phase 1 projects will have special needs for novel software. Public domain software is available at little or no cost to anyone who wants to use it, and these programs should be explored. In addition, such an archive would encourage the formation of neuroscience "news groups," or groups of users with similar interests, who could communicate by computer bulletin boards or electronic mail.

The committee recommends that an administrative structure be established to coordinate phase 1 activities. This Brain Map Advisory Panel (BMAP) should be composed of neuroscientists and computer and information scientists, with additional input from funding agency administrators. The panel would be responsible for the overall direction, evaluation, and coordination of consortia and for the development of necessary policies relating to establishment of a brain mapping effort. The committee also recommends that the Advisory Panel be responsible for consideration and development of editorial functions and policies relating to the ethical and sociological issues that will arise, including, but not limited to, correctness of information and quality control, intellectual property rights, rights to privacy, and freedom of information.

To develop the proper basis for a coordinated brain mapping effort, there must be communication among the consortia and some type of central oversight. The committee considered several mechanisms for providing such oversight and chose an advisory panel structure. The BMAP could also act as a clearinghouse for information and perform certain other functions:

- examine the needs of the entire neuroscience community;
- evaluate various aspects of database development including resource use, standards development, and effectiveness of incentives for data sharing;

- gather information from the consortia on emerging trends in the computer industry; and
- facilitate acceptance of the database among neuroscientists.

The BMAP should exercise oversight not in a top-down manner but as the result of communication between members of the consortia and the panel. This communication could occur through a variety of mechanisms including consortia representation on the panel and the sponsorship of regular meetings for consortia investigators. The panel should also coordinate establishment of the international registry of neuroscience databases and contacts and the archive of public domain software recommended by the committee. Finally, the panel should coordinate the Brain Mapping Initiative's interaction with funding agencies and with other, related scientific initiatives, and undertake the long-range planning of phase 2.

If electronic resources are to be accepted and utilized, scientists must be able to trust the accuracy of the information contained in the resource. One of the tasks of phase 1 investigators should be to begin to define mechanisms that ensure the appropriate use and labeling of different levels of data (from preliminary to peer-reviewed) and that allow for the deletion of information that becomes obsolete. In the committee's opinion, one of the best ways to achieve such goals is to develop edited archives and databases.

The committee recommends that the phase 1 and 2 projects of the Brain Mapping Initiative maintain a close relationship with the gene mapping and sequencing community and the Human Genome Project, and with other scientific computing efforts, including network initiatives such as NSFNET and the proposed National Research and Education Network. As part of these efforts, the committee further recommends that linkages be established with protein sequence and genome databases to enhance access to information about brain-specific genes.

The committee believes that the importance of gene mapping and sequencing to neuroscience should not be underestimated. In addition, much can be learned from existing database initiatives in this area, including the array of public and private databases that support the Human Genome Project and other established scientific networking efforts. Interaction with the ongoing scientific computing efforts in the global change research, astrophysics, and earth mapping communities would also be desirable.

The committee recommends that federal funding agencies develop requests for applications and/or cooperative agreements to support the formation of consortia and the activities of the Brain Map Advisory Panel. Limited use of contract mechanisms should also be considered when appropriate to the overall goals of the initiative.

The federal government uses several mechanisms to provide federal funds for research. One is contracts in which the government funds projects that its agencies propose, to be completed by an outside investigator according to a contract written by the government. Another mechanism, typical of NIH, ADAMHA, and NSF is grants to investigators or groups of investigators for research projects that are proposed, accomplished, and supervised by the investigators themselves. A third method, the cooperative agreement used by NSF, combines aspects of both grants and contracts. In the committee's opinion, the proposed Brain Mapping Initiative favors the use of grants because the development of usable resources should be intricately combined with the research itself. This kind of development is best carried out by scientists actively involved in neuroscience research.

The committee recommends that phases 1 and 2 of the Brain Mapping Initiative be international in scope and that they be funded by multiple sources in a coordinated fashion. The structure for administering the funding should ensure program stability and effectiveness. Possible funding structures include the identification of a lead agency or institute, or the establishment of formal administrative structures among two or more agencies.

The sources of neuroscience funding include the three institutes of ADAMHA and almost every institute of the NIH, as well as many other governmental agencies. The proposed organization of the Brain Mapping Initiative, especially the inclusion of an advisory panel and computer scientists, will not fit well into the usual funding structures administered by the NIH Division of Research Grants. To be successful, the proposed phase 1 projects require the involvement of multiple components of the federal biomedical research complex, as well as communication and cooperation among appropriate agencies of the Public Health Service, the Departments of Defense and Energy, and private foundations that fund biomedical science.

The committee concludes that the expected benefits of the proposed Brain Mapping Initiative justify the investment of necessary resources and recommends the appropriation

**of additional funding to support the establishment of phase
1 projects.**

The committee is sensitive to the current fiscal constraints now
being felt by the entire U.S. biomedical research effort and recognizes
the view held by many scientists that large-scale projects pose a threat
to the basic research enterprise. The committee believes, however,
that the Brain Mapping Initiative is an important project that should
be undertaken and that it could begin with an additional allocation
of approximately $10 million annually, with an overall evaluation to
occur at the end of five years. This investment represents only a
small part (less than 1 percent) of the entire U.S. neuroscience research effort, which is estimated to be more than $1.5 billion annually.
It is the committee's considered opinion that the success and probable
benefits of the initiative proposed here depend on and justify the
appropriation of this additional support.

Conclusion

It is clear that neuroscience stands at the threshold of a tremendous opportunity to unlock the mysteries of the brain and its functions.
Securing the benefits inherent in this opportunity requires a concerted,
interdisciplinary effort on the part of the many basic and clinical
neuroscientists engaged in research worldwide. It is equally clear
that this scientific enterprise is increasingly reliant on the use of sophisticated methodologies and computer technologies. The Brain
Mapping Initiative proposed in this report will allow investigators
studying the brain to view data in new ways, to communicate data to
each other more efficiently, and to access data from any of the neuroscience subspecialties. So enabled, neuroscientists will be able to map
the brain and its functions, thus realizing the full potential of the
electronic resources now available to the scientific enterprise and en-
suring that society will receive the greatest possible benefits from
neuroscience research.

Note

1. These species are intended as starting points. The committee also recognizes the
need to include data from other, vertebrate and invertebrate, species.

1

Introduction

The computer, the instrument of the sciences of complexity, will reveal a new cosmos never before perceived. Because of its ability to manage and process enormous quantities of information in a reliable, mechanical way, the computer, as a scientific research tool, has already revealed a new universe. This universe was previously inaccessible, not because it was so small or so far away, but because it was so complex that no human mind could disentangle it.

HEINZ PAGELS, *Dreams of Reason*

Scientists studying the brain have generated a wealth of experimental data, and this explosion of information has unlocked many of the secrets of brain functioning. Moreover, this progress already has helped to alleviate some of the human suffering that results from brain injury and disease. Ironically, however, the field is threatened by its own success in that the sheer mass of information available to basic and clinical neuroscientists is becoming unmanageable. Effective access to existing neuroscience information is critical to the enterprise of discovery: such information forms the basis for new hypotheses, drives the search for improved methodology, and, ultimately, leads to the advances necessary for fundamental improvements in human health.

One way to improve access and speed the meaningful dissemination of scientific discoveries is through the application of sophisticated computer and information-sharing technologies. These enabling

21

technologies currently assist space exploration, earth mapping, global communication, and dissection of the atom, among other functions. In certain types of scientific investigation, computer and information technologies have led directly to new ways of observing, simulating, and manipulating biological and physical processes. The neuroscience community has seen an escalation in the use of computer technologies to collect and analyze data, organize the data of individual investigators, and share experimental results with other researchers. As computer-based tools for three-dimensional representations, simulation and modeling, and storage of large data sets improve, their usefulness to the study of the brain becomes more apparent. During the past decade, many neuroscientists have become interested in the expanded application of computer and information technologies in their research, with the goal of forging new pathways for communication among investigators and managing diverse collections of scientific information.

This report results from the deliberations of the Institute of Medicine's Committee on a National Neural Circuitry Database, whose objective was to consider the desirability, feasibility, and possible ways of implementing a family of electronic (e.g., networks) and digital (e.g., computer databases) resources for the enhancement of neuroscience research. The committee was formed in response to a request from Lewis Judd, director of the National Institute of Mental Health (NIMH); it was funded by NIMH in cooperation with the National Institute on Drug Abuse (NIDA) and the National Science Foundation (NSF). The impetus for the study came in large part from the need expressed by neuroscientists for new ways of collecting and integrating the large amount of data they generate. An additional motivation was the increased attention of the general scientific community and of policymakers regarding the challenges presented by these emerging technologies and their potential to support and improve research. Initiatives such as the National Research and Education Network, proposed by Senator Albert Gore and supported by the President's Science Advisor, and the long-range plans of the National Library of Medicine to construct digital libraries are examples of this increased attention.

The incorporation of computer and information technology into a scientific field often begins through trial and error, driven by individual scientists who respond to opportunities as they emerge. The initial use of these technologies is often highly individual, and it generally proceeds in the absence of any coordination within specific scientific disciplines. As usage expands, however, the need for coordination and standardization increases, raising important questions about the development of appropriate governmental policies, which ultimately affect the conduct of research both nationally and internationally.

Within this broad context, the charge to this committee was to

- formulate a position on the requirements for and appropriateness of establishing a family of digital resources for basic and clinical neuroscience that would allow optimal data communication and sharing among investigators;
- consider the scope and elements of data that should constitute these resources and determine strategies for representing the diverse data types generated by neuroscientists;
- examine existing national databases to identify successful data storage, retrieval, and sharing strategies as well as potential pitfalls for the establishment of computerized resources for neuroscience;
- describe an effective structure for a family of computerized resources to allow its efficient establishment and optimal coordination for use by the neuroscience research community, clinical investigators, clinicians, students, and educators; and
- provide recommendations on future directions in program development for NIMH, NIDA, and NSF with respect to such computerized resources.

To fulfill its charge, the committee drew on many sources of expertise, beginning with the experience and knowledge of its members. A diverse set of activities supplemented the committee's deliberations and provided key data for the study. Between October 1989 and October 1990, the committee convened four task forces, in total, comprising 43 neuroscientists and computer and information science experts, that considered various resource options in terms of varied levels of neuroscience inquiry (see Appendix A). The committee also solicited input from the neuroscience community through published requests for opinions, letters to the present officers and past presidents of the Society for Neuroscience, and a series of three symposia and open hearings (these activities are summarized in Appendixes B and C).

Based on these activities and deliberations, this report focuses on the benefits that could be realized by the successful application of electronic and digital resources to the conduct of research into brain functions. The report's recommendations provide a structural framework for initiating a program to apply these resources; they also identify certain key elements that should be considered by those who may be charged with implementing such a program. Thus, the report should be useful for policymakers and directors of institutions who will be involved in the endeavor. It is hoped that the committee's findings will underscore for this audience the importance of increasing the integration of information technology and computer science with neuroscience in particular and with the biomedical research enterprise in general. In addition, the report is aimed toward working scientists to foster an understanding of the benefits to be gained by using these resources in their own research and by sharing their results. As we enter the Decade of the Brain, the committee believes that an exciting opportunity exists to harness computer and information technology for the enhancement of neuroscience research. The advantages to be derived from seizing this opportunity include accelerated progress in understanding and treating neurological and mental illness, brain and spinal cord injury, and developmental deficits.

2

Advancing Neuroscience
in the Decade of the Brain

Not very long ago, the feasibility of mapping the distinguishable regions of the human brain in relation to their functional roles seemed remote. With the tremendous advances in neuroscience in the past two decades, however, the opportunity now exists to approach the integrated understanding of brain structure and functioning necessary to clarify the neurobiological basis of human thought and emotion and to discern the mechanisms that underlie sensory perception and locomotor functions. Many of the intricate anatomical connections of the brain are being defined in great detail. New capabilities have emerged to identify and describe the biochemical, molecular, and genetic mechanisms that determine brain structure and functions. The activity of the human brain during mental activity can be measured and visualized. It is even becoming possible to monitor simultaneously the activity of many neurons within complex neural networks during discrete behaviors. The challenge now is to establish a comprehensive initiative that will increase the ability of neuroscientists to make discoveries about the brain and to apply this knowledge to the many mental and neurological disorders that affect humankind.

The progress made in this area has occurred primarily through the concerted efforts of increasing numbers of individual investigators, working mostly in small groups on highly specific projects. The body of information gained through such efforts has grown in a piecemeal fashion; it has now reached a point of limitation, in terms of its usefulness, because the mass of information is so great and its dissemination so poorly coordinated that critical data are often difficult to recover and define. Indeed, this approach to neuroscience research, which was so successful in the past, may soon limit advances in the same way that a single surveyor who charts a field cannot hope to map a continent without a coordinated plan involving other mappers. A Brain Mapping Initiative could identify those aspects of information exchange infrastructure that are critical to addressing a broader goal, one that will include the advantages of single-investigator projects and yet also yield the benefits of a larger, coordinated program. The Brain Mapping Initiative is intended to subsume all the proposed aspects of a National Neural Circuitry Database outlined in the charge to this committee. It is also designed to express explicitly the goals of the proposed effort and reflect more adequately the complex of electronic and digital resources that will be required.

A consensus is emerging that the initial steps can now be taken toward the global task of understanding brain structure and functioning. The impact of digital computer technology began in the physical sciences three or four decades ago and led to such current large-scale efforts as the supercollider, space telescope, and interplanetary probes. In neuroscience, the increasing availability of new enabling technologies is likely to have similar, far-reaching impacts. The development of high-density memory chips and the latest generation of microprocessors provides a key stimulus to accelerated development of image analysis graphics and image manipulation—a set of capabilities known as visualization computing (McCormick et al., 1987). The emergence of parallel processing, scientific visualization workstations, and high-capacity digital communications may provide the technical support needed to conduct coordinated projects in neuroscience.

A comprehensive, coordinated effort to understand basic organizational patterns of brain connections needs to be undertaken. This effort should include a definition of the chemical identity of neuronal populations and a description of neuronal structure and neuronal circuit organization in each region in sufficient detail to clarify the computational processes involved. The pace of future advances in neuroscience will depend on critical choices, which need to be made now, regarding the handling of information to be gathered in the future. At issue is whether neuroscientists will embark on a large-scale effort to develop and integrate new forms of technology for acquiring and managing information.

Complexity and the Need for Information Management

The brain exhibits by far the greatest complexity of any of the organs of the human body. Indeed, there is reason to believe that a substantial percentage of the human genome plays a role in creating neural structure, connectional patterns, and neurochemistry. The brain's responsibilities are numerous and include initiation of movement, mediation of sensation, and regulation of other body organs. Its functioning provides the basis of perception and cognition and underlies emotion and creative expression. Although described as a master computer, the brain is fundamentally more complex and its processes far more subtle than those of any current computer design. With the advantage of parallel operation of neuronal populations, the brain manages and controls a wide variety of tasks simultaneously, reliably, and with rapid precision. Indeed, much of the brain's work proceeds even in the absence of an individual's conscious awareness.

All brain activity results from electrical and chemical communication among neurons (the primary signaling cells of the brain), each of which can communicate with other neurons using signals at rates of up to 1,000 events (impulses) per second. To understand the brain, neuroscientists must measure and analyze the rapid changes in neuronal signaling activity that occur over the vast networks of cells and connections. The scope of this endeavor is immense. It is estimated that the human brain contains more than 100 billion neurons, and each neuron maintains an average of about 1,000 connections, called synapses, with other neurons. Some neurons have as many as 200,000 synapses. During each moment of daily life, neural signals may be transmitted across any of approximately 100 trillion synapses.

Improvements in human health require greater integration and synthesis of knowledge than can be gained simply by describing the intricate, extensive circuitry that characterizes a normal or average brain. To treat schizophrenia, Alzheimer's disease, brain injury, degenerative diseases, developmental deficits, and chemical dependency, it will be necessary to understand the biochemical reactions and specialized neurochemistry expressed by different types of neurons. In addition, neuroscience must take into account the differences among individuals that arise from environmental as well as hereditary factors. Such differences range from subtle genetic variations in small populations of neurons to differing developmental states and wide-ranging perturbations of major brain systems.

In many ways, because of the brain's organization, neuroscience research is obliged to proceed along a multilevel hierarchy, from behavior to molecular interactions (see Chapter 3). Each level of research uses numerous techniques that are specifically designed to collect information appropriate to that level. But information from one level often has important implications for knowledge at other levels. Effective synthesis of the data depends on the traditional academic skills of the scholar; it is becoming increasingly difficult, however, for neuro-scientists to identify, manage, and process all the information needed for the efficient design and conduct of their research. Even with well-developed traditional academic skills, the neuroscientist clearly needs new information organization and access technologies. Electronic information management provides assistance at a high level of syn-thesis—in much the same way that hand calculators and word pro-cessors facilitate tasks like balancing a budget or creating a document.

To draw an analogy, neuroscientists are like puzzle builders who must integrate and fit together numerous small pieces of information derived from the hundreds of available techniques. Metaphorically, the challenge is to assemble a multimillion-piece, three-dimensional puzzle, starting with an incomplete set of pieces (many key facts about the brain remain unknown) and incomplete knowledge of how different pieces relate to one another (seemingly disparate facts are often closely related). In addition, the puzzle that represents the brain must depict more than simply a structure. It must integrate structure with function, function with chemistry, and chemistry with genetic mechanisms. Generating the data that represent the individual pieces of the puzzle is difficult in and of itself: the techniques available to neuroscientists all have inherent limitations and usually produce only incremental bits of information, although every year more bits are added and new puzzle pieces identified. The next decade is expected to provide enough new pieces to allow for the discovery of exciting new ways to understand, protect, and restore brain functioning. But innovative methods of information assembly and integration will be as important as the discovery of the individual pieces.

In science, the conventional way to gain access to relevant infor-mation generated outside one's own laboratory is through the study of scientific literature and by formal and informal communication with other scientists. As the number of publications and literature sources grows, the use of such resources becomes more and more expensive, inefficient, and incomplete. It now takes an inordinate amount of time to sift through the various conventional publications. The process usually requires a narrowly focused search strategy, which yields less information than is actually available. Eventually, the process is self limiting. To pursue the puzzle analogy, it is like try-ing to assemble the three-dimensional puzzle by using two-dimen-sional sketches of the pieces, rather than being able to hold the origi-nal three-dimensional pieces. Furthermore, because the pieces are scattered in various locations, most of one's time is spent in looking for the individual pieces and not in trying to understand how they are interrelated.

For many years, a number of neuroscientists have envisioned alternative strategies for coping with the problem of information management, which is distinct from that of acquiring more data. Information management is aimed toward realizing the greatest benefit from the data that already exist. Two major kinds of information management are the most critical for neuroscience: (1) databases, which allow at least partial automation of the task of relating diverse data types in a systematic, efficient manner, and (2) the capacity for visualization of structures in three dimensions. Visualization computing, whether by machine or by the scholar's brain, captures the discoverable architecture of the brain and relates this architecture to brain functioning.

Scientists mapping the human genome or sequencing biologically important proteins have been using databases for years (Smith, 1990; Vela, 1990). These databases contain precise information, obtained directly from experimental investigation, regarding the sequence of base pairs of specific genes, their locations on specific chromosomes, and the amino acid sequences of known and newly discovered proteins. Investigators consider these databases invaluable for a host of reasons. Most commonly, researchers check a newly charted protein sequence against thousands of other known sequences to see if their new sequence is related to other known proteins. Similarly, the base pair sequences of genes of one species are routinely checked against sequences from other species to determine the level of homology of specific genes across species. Beyond simple comparison, knowledge of base pairs and protein sequences can provide key information regarding biological functions. Thus, protein and gene mapping databases are more than simply references; they are quickly becoming essential components of the scientific process of discovery (see Box 2-1; DeLisi, 1988; Colwell, 1989).

The experience of the protein and gene mapping community is an instructive example of the benefits to be gained from incorporating database and information technology into biomedical research efforts. There are major differences, however, that must be taken into account when considering how to extend this approach to the field of neuroscience. Chief among these differences is that of complexity. Although proteins exhibit tremendous diversity, much of this diversity is represented by the linear sequence of amino acids that make up each protein. Such linear arrays are easy to store in traditional databases and also represent the key information for genes. All proteins also have a three-dimensional structure, however. Computerized molecular modeling has been very successful in displaying molecular structures in three dimensions (Howard Hughes Medical Institute, 1990), but it is not yet possible to incorporate these three-dimensional models into

---

BOX 2-1 THE GENE FOR NEUROFIBROMATOSIS 1

First described in the late nineteenth century, neurofibromatosis 1 (NF1) is an inherited condition affecting 1 in every 3,500 people. The two most common symptoms of NF1 are areas of dark pigmentation on the skin, and benign but often disfiguring tumors, called neurofibromas, beneath the skin. A wide range of other, less common symptoms appear in connection with NF1, and these include learning disabilities, mental retardation, malignancies of the nervous system, scoliosis, and other bone abnormalities.

In 1987, James Gusella and his colleagues at Massachusetts General Hospital (Seizinger et al., 1987) and Ray White and his research team at the University of Utah (Barker et al., 1987), localized the gene responsible for causing NF1 to chromosome 17. The abnormal gene was subsequently isolated and sequenced by White's team and by Francis Collins and his coworkers at the University of Michigan (Lewis, 1990). The next step was to translate the genetic code into an amino acid sequence, which was then fed into a computer and matched against databases of other known sequences. Similarities were found between the protein sequence of NF1 and those of two other genes, one being a gene that codes for a group of proteins called GAP proteins, which are thought to suppress tumor growth, and the other being a tumor-suppressing gene in yeast. The homologies seem logical—altered GAP protein function could certainly have manifestations similar to those observed in NF1. Although many important details remain to be filled in, what scientists already know about GAP proteins and yeast genes will provide a springboard for researchers striving to understand neurofibromatosis.

The knowledge base established by White, Collins, Gusella, and their colleagues is likely to attract researchers from many disciplines that have not traditionally studied neurofibromatosis—cancer researchers in particular, because NF1 now joins the growing list of potential tumor-suppressor genes. A complete solution to the NF1 puzzle is unlikely in the very near future, but discovery of the NF1 gene and its protein product promises to speed development of prenatal diagnosis of and possibly treatment for NF1.

---

traditional databases. In contrast to molecular biology, understanding the diversity inherent in brain structure and functioning requires the three-dimensional display of many types of experimental information. Because the fundamental complexity of neuroscience data exceeds that of molecular biology data, the development of information management technologies to enhance neuroscience research will present great challenges. Yet such challenges are approachable, and the potential benefits to greater understanding of the human brain are compelling reasons for confronting them.

Examples of the Value of Integrating Knowledge to Solve Problems

Achieving advances in neuroscience is a difficult task, particularly those advances that yield improvements in the treatment and understanding of neurological, developmental, and mental diseases. Integration of knowledge across the areas of investigation at each level of the neural hierarchy is required. The importance of applying these diverse methodologies to discern how the brain functions can be illustrated by the following explicit examples of the hierarchical organization within neuroscience (see also Chapter 3).

Vision: How we see affects how we think

The visual system, one of the most intensively studied systems of the brain, reveals remarkable complexity in organization and functioning. Because it occurs so effortlessly, vision is something we often take for granted and consider to be a fairly simple matter. In fact, however, the brain conducts extensive processing of all visual information to allow for pattern recognition, interpretation, and appreciation of such concepts as beauty. The neural underpinnings of these abilities are contained within a rich, intricate network of pathways that involve billions of individual neurons. The system also includes muscles and motor regions of the brain to point the eyes toward areas of interest and to track objects in motion (see Box 2-2).

Investigations of the visual system have used a wide range of techniques that have contributed substantial knowledge regarding the anatomy, biochemistry, and physiology of the system. The information that reaches the eyes is first processed by a thin layer of cells that make up the retina at the back of the eye. Through exquisitely sensitive signal transduction mechanisms, retinal cells respond to a range of inputs, including color. Coordination among the cells in the retina also provides the first filtering of incoming information by the balancing of excitatory and inhibitory processes. From the retina, information is transmitted to a pair of nuclei on each side of the brain, called the lateral geniculate nuclei, in a highly ordered pattern so that each half of the visual field is precisely mapped onto the lateral geniculate on the opposite side of the brain. So well understood is this map that differing kinds of visual deficits can indicate the exact location of damage (a frequent occurrence following stroke or as a result of the pressure of a growing tumor) along the pathways of the visual system. The lateral geniculate nuclei relay visual information to the primary visual cortex. Again, the information is mapped in a highly ordered pattern with segregation of the inputs from each eye.

BOX 2-2 SOMETIMES THE BRAIN LEARNS
TO IGNORE VISUAL INPUT

To focus on objects in the visual field, the muscles of both eyes are normally coordinated so that both eyes move in unison. But abnormal eye muscle development in one eye can cause misalignment of the two eyes, often resulting in a condition known as *strabismus*. A child born with this condition will favor one eye to avoid double vision, and, over time, visual acuity in the less favored eye deteriorates. Left uncorrected, the child becomes blind in that eye. Before the neural basis of binocular vision was understood, procedures to correct strabismus were typically done at age 8 or 9, long after permanent deterioration had occurred. Today, the condition is corrected very early to protect such children's normal vision.

Measurement of how neurons in the visual cortex respond to different stimuli has revealed much about the microprocessing of information. Most important, many visual neurons are selective for specific features in the visual world. For example, Nobel laureates David Hubel and Torsten Wiesel discovered that many neurons are selective for the orientation of a bar, which allows them to signal the presence of particular edges and contours (Hubel and Wiesel, 1979). Since their discovery, other researchers have described types of neurons that are sensitive to color, directional movements, and, at higher levels, even complex shapes like faces.

From the primary visual cortex, information is transmitted to many other cortical areas involved in higher aspects of visual processing. This dispersion of information is necessary for all the activities associated with vision, including reading, writing, and recognition of objects in the environment. The monkey has 32 regions of the cortex that are known to be involved in some type of visual processing (Plate 2-1). Each of these regions subserves a specific function; yet they are interlinked by more than 300 separate pathways. Much visual information ultimately reaches neural centers involved in cognitive functions and emotions. Understanding these parallel, distributed pathways has important implications for understanding the deficits from brain injury, including stroke. They also help explain some of the most puzzling aspects of these problems. (For example, some stroke patients can recognize words and objects such as tables and chairs, but cannot recognize a loved one's face [Sacks, 1970]. Because each of these different stimuli present distinct features, damage to one area of the cortex may affect the perception of one constellation of features but not others.)

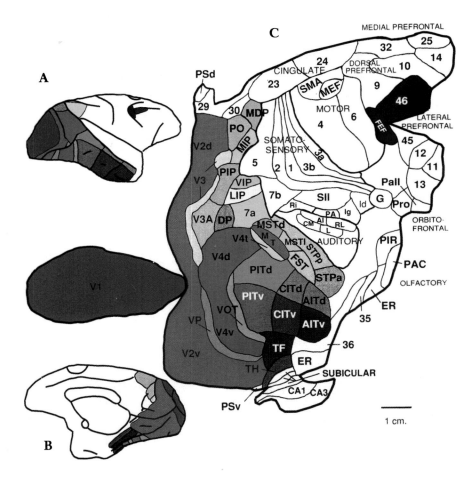

PLATE 2-1 Maps of the monkey cerebral cortex, with the visual processing region shaded. **A** and **B** are two-dimensional representations of the cerebral cortex from different perspectives. **C** is a two-dimensional map of an "un-folded" cortex, in which topological relationships are preserved and areal distortions kept to a minimum. This map was generated manually from the contours through a series of histological sections. Figure courtesy of David Van Essen, Division of Biology, California Institute of Technology.

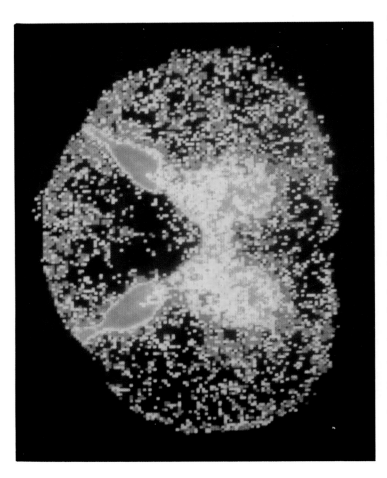

PLATE 2-2 Opiate receptor localization in spinal cord by autoradiography. High densities of opiate receptors (dark orange) are found in the dorsal horn, an area associated with pain perception. Autoradiographic imaging is useful for exploring sites of drug action and for understanding how drugs exert their effects. Image courtesy of Michael J. Kuhar, Neuroscience Branch, National Institute of Drug Abuse Addiction Research Center.

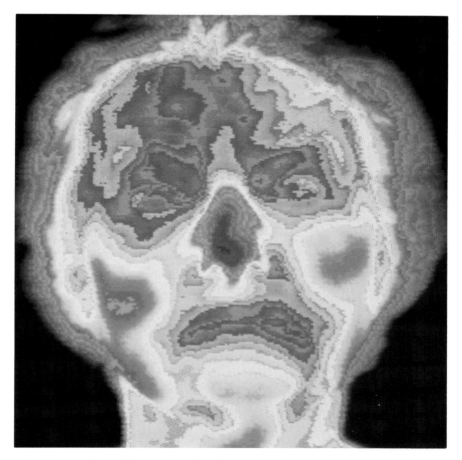

PLATE 2-3 Infrared thermograph of a patient with post-herpetic neuralgia, a condition involving persistent pain in areas affected by a herpes zoster infection at least three months after healing of the skin lesions. Areas of pathological pain are associated with increased skin temperature (red represents highest skin temperature). Figure reprinted from Rowbotham and Fields, 1989, with permission from Elsevier Science Publishers.

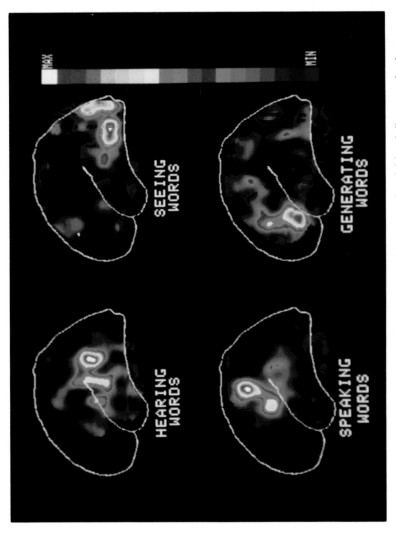

PLATE 3-1 Computerized PET images showing the changes in local blood flow in the brain, associated with local changes in neuronal activity, that occur during different states of information processing. Image courtesy of Marcus Raichle, Department of Neurology, Washington University School of Medicine.

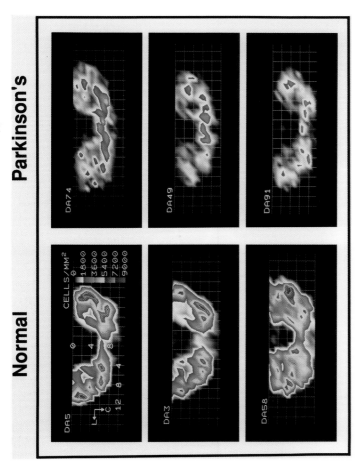

PLATE 3-2 Cell frequency maps illustrating the regional distribution of midbrain dopaminergic neurons in three normal and three parkinsonian brains. The colored areas represent regions that contain different frequencies of cells (e.g., white areas contain 1-1,800 cells per square millimeter (cells/mm2) and red areas contain 7,201-9,000 cells/mm2). The higher frequencies of cells are markedly reduced within the substantia nigra in the three parkinsonian brains. Reprinted from German et al., 1989, with permission from *Annals of Neurology*.

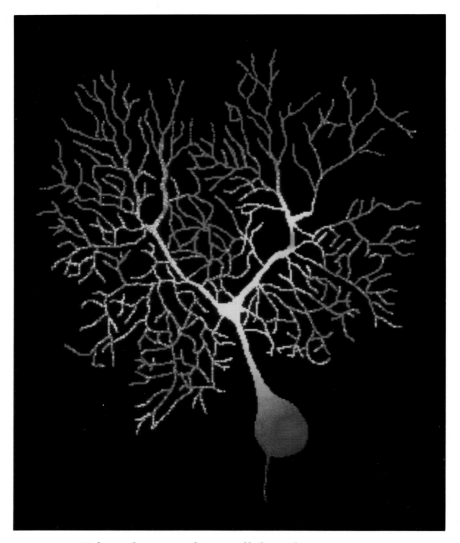

PLATE 3-3 False color map of intracellular calcium concentration in a guinea pig cerebellar Purkinje cell at the onset of a wave of complex spike activity. A high calcium concentration is observed in the outer portions of the dendritic tree. The map was produced from microfluorometric imaging of the fluorescent calcium indicator fura-2. Image courtesy of D.W. Tank and J. A. Connor, Molecular Biophysics Department, AT&T Bell Laboratories, Murray Hill, NJ; M. Sugimori and R. R. Llinas, Department of Physiology and Biophysics, New York University School of Medicine, New York, NY. Reprinted with permission of *Science*.

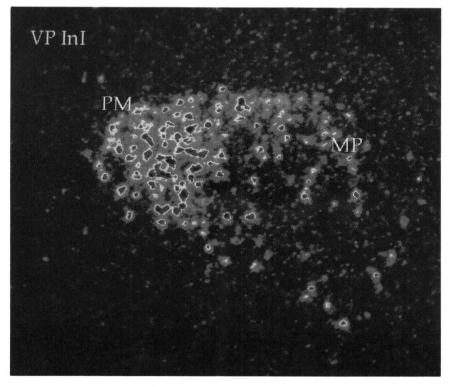

PLATE 3-4 Computer-enhanced image of vasopressin heteronuclear RNA in the hypothalamic paraventricular nucleus (PVN), as revealed by in situ hybridization utilizing a probe directed against vasopressin intronic (VP InI) gene sequences. The image is derived from an autoradiograph and demonstrates expression of the VP gene in functionally distinct divisions of the PVN (posterior magnocellular (PM) and medial parvocellular (MP) regions). Intronic in situ hybridization allows localization of short-lived heteronuclear RNA at the cellular level, and in combination with computer-based image analytic procedures can reveal rapid stimulus-induced changes in gene expression in discrete neuronal populations. Image provided by James P. Herman and Stanley J. Watson, Mental Health Research Institute, The University of Michigan.

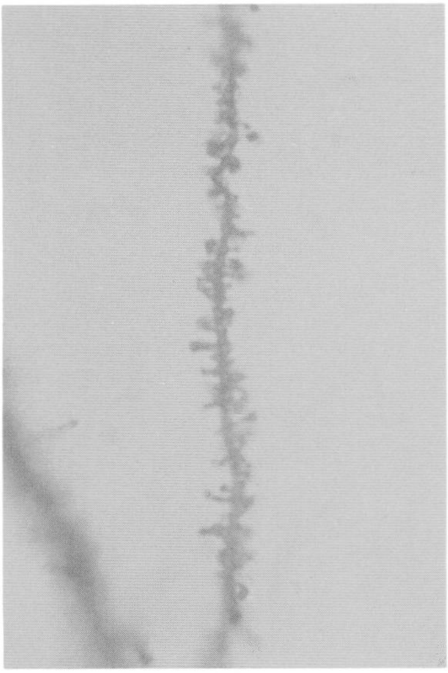

PLATE 3-5 Photomicrographs of dendrites from the brains of a **A**, a young animal, and **B**, an aged animal. The extensions from the main dendritic shaft are dendritic "spines." Note the thinning of dendritic spines in the aged brain. **C**. Color-enhanced freeze-fracture of a single dendritic spine. Photomicrographs courtesy of Fidia Pharmaceutical Corporation.

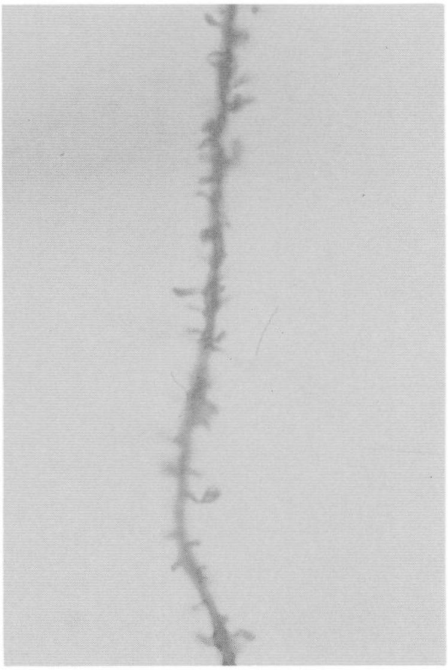

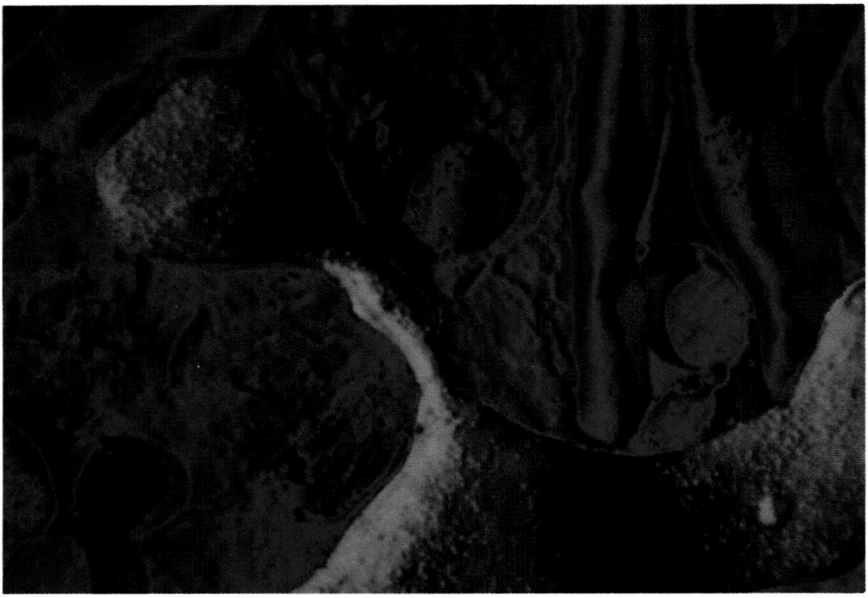

Cognition and recognition are not the only results of visual sensation. The retina also projects visual information to nuclei that are involved not in feature analysis but in controlling the eye muscles. These pathways mediate the turning of the eyes in the direction of a stimulus; the coordinated, simultaneous movement of both eyes; and the ability to track moving objects in the visual field. Again, certain kinds of damage affect these pathways and may result in debilitating deficits.

As in all neural systems, the functioning of the visual system relies on the coordinated activity of neurons that communicate with each other using electrical and chemical signals generated by hundreds of different molecules, including neurotransmitters, second messengers, and signal transduction molecules. Many of these molecules have been found in distinctive patterns in specific areas of the visual system. The combination of complex physiological responses, complex anatomical pathways, and hundreds of neurochemical interactions creates a system that is extremely difficult to disentangle. Despite all the information we possess, we still do not understand the fundamental nature of visual perception, nor do we understand the specific computations carried out in the vast networks at each stage of information processing.

Finding answers to these challenging questions will require not only additional experimental data but new strategies for assembling the available information to facilitate integration of the diverse data types. To accomplish this integration, the use of three-dimensional graphics, sophisticated database technology, and greater levels of electronic communication among investigators will be critical. For example, maps of the anatomical pathways must be overlaid with neurochemical maps to understand how the wide repertoire of chemical modulatory influences may be related to different aspects of visual perception and visual-motor coordination. Computer simulations and realistic computational models, based on physiological and anatomical data, are needed to understand the specific signal-processing strategies used in various regions of the visual system. Such computational studies are also of interest to engineers and computer scientists in the construction of new types of sensors and signal detectors for nonbiological uses.

It is clear that the full potential of visual system research has yet to be realized. Progress in this field will contribute to the ability to treat or compensate for visual deficits caused by brain injury. In addition, this work can contribute to the amelioration of blindness and diseases of the visual system, including glaucoma, diabetic retinopathy, and inherited retinal degenerations. The mapping and physiological characterization of the multiple visual system pathways also have direct relevance for understanding other portions of the brain, especially other portions of the cerebral cortex.

Substance abuse: The search for the biology of self-destruction

A large fraction of the U.S. population uses substances that are injurious to personal health. These substances range from legally approved drugs (e.g., nicotine and alcohol) to illegal drugs (e.g., cocaine and heroin) that are accompanied by grave societal costs such as violent crime and infant mortality. The key to understanding and dealing with substance abuse lies in the brain. One path of research has already led to the critically important discovery that there are cell-surface receptors not only for neurotransmitters but also for many drugs, including nicotine, marijuana, heroin and other opiate drugs, and benzodiazepines, such as the tranquilizer Valium® (Plate 2-2). Often, certain drugs bind to the same receptor to which a particular neurotransmitter binds. For example, the two kinds of acetylcholine receptors were first distinguished by the fact that one bound nicotine and the other did not. Such receptors have been mapped to specific nuclei of the brain. Thus, the notion that certain drugs have specific actions in discrete brain regions offers a possible route for disrupting the effects of those drugs.

But the problem goes much deeper. For example, alcohol does not act at specific receptor sites; its effects are much more general throughout the brain. Furthermore, all psychoactive substances produce experiences that provide some type of motivation or pleasure that can lead to addiction. Therefore, addiction to medically harmful substances is directly related to the involvement of brain systems that mediate the normal pleasurable experiences associated with many day-to-day activities such as eating, drinking, and socialization. Neuroscientists do not completely understand the location, organization, and chemistry of the system in the brain that underlies positive emotions and pleasure and, with that, the pleasurable, motivating effects of drugs and alcohol. Certain fascinating clues, however, have been found. For example, animals will self-administer cocaine so avidly that they totally ignore food; yet this behavior can be completely reversed if the neurotransmitter dopamine is removed from an area of the brain known as the nucleus accumbens. No conceptual framework similar to those that guide our understanding of the visual and motor systems has emerged to explain this phenomenon. Many scientists hypothesize that a number of brain regions in the limbic system and hypothalamus are involved, but the connections between these regions are extremely complex and not well understood.

Two types of databases could greatly enhance research into the biology of substance abuse. Databases that allow for the easy comparison of brain distribution patterns of receptors for the many substances that are abused would be invaluable. Their usefulness would be particularly great if distribution patterns could be compared with the known circuitry of the brain, with the associated distribution patterns of known neurotransmitters, receptors, and ion channels, and with the results of behavioral studies related to the neural mechanisms of addiction. No conventional library system currently allows for this level of analysis of visual material. A second, related kind of database would contain information about the known neural pathways implicated in addiction. Such a resource could aid the development of a viable picture of the brain system involved in mediating the reinforcing aspects of drug use and in the formulation of efficient strategies for research into areas where more information is needed. Substance abuse offers a compelling example of how the availability of comprehensive databases that incorporate and integrate information from many fields, including chemical neuroanatomy, pharmacology, and biopsychology, would almost certainly speed the development of effective treatments for a widespread, serious threat to human health.

Pain: Sometimes a warning, sometimes a curse

Pain is a ubiquitous reality of life. We need pain to recognize sprained ankles, overstressed back muscles, kidney stones, infections, and a host of other ills. This useful warning system can go awry, however, and become an intractable barrier to a happy, productive life (Plate 2-3). The neural underpinnings of pain involve almost every region of the brain, spinal cord, and peripheral nervous system. Moreover, these neural mechanisms interact with other systems of the body, including the immune system and certain endocrine glands, and are even affected by changes in the metabolic status of the individual (e.g., as in diabetes). Pain is thus a remarkably complex process about which much remains to be learned.

In its simplest form, pain results from the activation of peripheral nerves by certain types of stimuli impinging on the skin and internal organs. This neural information is transmitted to and processed by specific parts of the spinal cord. From the spinal cord, information about injury is transmitted to numerous brain regions, including specific relay nuclei that, in turn, transmit it to the sensory part of the cerebral cortex and to nonspecific nuclei that disperse the information through their abundant connections to other brain regions. Information regarding a painful stimulus reaches brain regions that are involved in emotion, sensory perception, body movement, and hormonal release. In addition, the information reaches brain regions that connect back to the spinal cord and that are capable of modulating the activity of spinal neurons. These complex connections form the anatomical basis for systems that can activate or inhibit pain. The pain system also utilizes scores of different neurotransmitters and an interesting group of peptides that include endorphin and enkephalin, which are similar to morphine.

The intricacy of these connections explains in part some of the most fascinating and worrisome aspects of pain perception. For example, it is common for wounded people to walk considerable distances to reach help without conscious awareness of their pain and for people with malignant cancerous growths to be free of pain in the cancer's early stages (possibly because of the activation of pain-inhibiting systems). On the other hand, people who have had amputations, including mastectomy, often feel pain in the amputated body part, despite its absence (possibly because of pain-activating systems). The intricacy of the pain system also accounts for the wide variety of kinds of pain people experience, of kinds of treatments that are effective, and of scientific and clinical disciplines that deal with pain.

The need for enhanced communication in neuroscientific disciplines is well illustrated by the example of pain research and treatment. In the clinical arena, neurosurgeons have had a long-standing interest in finding ways to disrupt appropriate brain areas to alleviate intractable pain. The electrical stimulation or selective destruction of such areas has met with limited success, sometimes utter failure; in the worst-case scenario, the pain returns and is greater than before the surgery. Further advances in these and other techniques depend on expansion of knowledge from anatomical, electrophysiological, and neurochemical studies in animals.

The experience and knowledge of other disciplines are also important. For example, anesthesiologists deal with pain on an everyday basis, but the responsibility for pain management typically changes from the anesthesiologist to other health care providers as a patient is moved from the recovery or delivery room to a regular medical/surgical ward. As a result, widely divergent strategies are used. Increased communication among these various care providers could lead to more effective pain management and the ability to use pain (and the lack of it) as a diagnostic tool. As it becomes clearer that pain management has a substantial impact on recovery following surgery, communication between health care providers and basic researchers should be increased to promote better information transfer.

Basic pain research has generated an impressive amount of knowledge about the brain and the way it deals with pain. Recent work has begun to characterize the connectivity patterns of spinal and brainstem pathways that mediate pain, as well as their biochemical and physiological qualities. It is becoming increasingly evident that the neural mechanisms underlying musculoskeletal, cutaneous (skin), and visceral (internal organs) pain are different, and these differences are under active investigation. Differences in chronic and acute pain also are being intensely studied. Investigators are defining as well the actions of various immune system products at the site of injury and their contribution to pain. A very recent development has been the use of animal models for pain caused by arthritis and peripheral nerve injury. This work has brought the first hints that damage to the nerves can result in permanent changes in the spinal cord, and possibly in other brain regions, that may well be responsible for intractable pain syndromes. Prevention of these changes by early intervention may help to alleviate a sizable proportion of the human suffering that results from this kind of pain.

Given the prevalence of pain and the societal burdens it imposes, there is a pressing need to find better ways to transfer into clinical practice what is being learned from basic research and to apply clinical observations to the design of basic research experiments. A family of computerized resources could promote these information transfers by making anatomical, biochemical, and physiological data available in a manner that integrates the information graphically, cross-references data from other disciplines, and provides relevant clinical observations. A repository for various pain diagnostic and treatment strategies and observed outcomes would also be useful. Finding answers to the many unresolved questions about pain and its varied pathologies will depend, in part, on several communication-related factors including the most efficient use of the information that exists now and the widest dissemination of the information that will be generated in the future.

Schizophrenia: Broken minds, shattered dreams

For the 2 million Americans who suffer from schizophrenia, the world is often terrifying, confusing, and bitterly lonely. This devastating disease of the brain most often strikes people in adolescence and young adulthood and is expressed in a variety of forms, depending on the specific constellation of symptoms that occur. These forms range from those with predominantly "negative" (loss of function) symptoms to those with mainly "positive" symptoms (exaggerated or distorted brain functions). Thus, a person with schizophrenia will exhibit some combination of the following: hallucinations and delusions, blunted or inappropriate emotional expression, inability to derive pleasure from normal experiences, cognitive difficulties, and abnormal socialization. Major efforts are under way in neuroscience to discover the causes of schizophrenia, to understand the mechanisms of the disease, and to find better treatments for those whose lives are burdened by this illness.

Researchers are pursuing three major areas of investigation: neurochemical abnormalities, structural and functional brain abnormalities, and possible genetic and environmental causes of the disease. The discovery that certain drugs can alleviate the hallucinations and delusions of schizophrenics provided strong evidence that a neurochemical imbalance was important in the disease. Because all effective drugs were found to decrease the effects of the neurotransmitter dopamine, research is now focusing on the mechanisms of dopamine action in the brain and on mapping the areas of the brain that use dopamine in neural transmission. Unlike Parkinson's disease, a condition in which a specific group of dopamine-containing neurons die, people with schizophrenia have no single, well-defined area of the brain that is damaged; rather, anatomical studies suggest that many dopamine-containing brain areas are affected. In addition, unlike Parkinson's disease, which exhibits a loss of dopamine owing to neuronal death, schizophrenia displays an apparent excess of dopamine activity. This excess activity may be due to an abnormally high number of a specific type of cell-surface receptor for dopamine, the D_2 receptor. (Receptor subtypes are themselves a subject of intense interest because each subtype behaves differently; thus, their existence adds ever deeper levels of complexity to the questions regarding the precise role of dopamine in schizophrenia.)

Further research is necessary to understand how abnormalities in the dopamine system of the brain contribute to the symptoms of schizophrenia. Evidence is mounting that other neurotransmitters are also involved. For example, it is well known that dopamine blocking drugs are effective only against the positive symptoms of schizophrenia, which suggests that the blunting of affect and other negative symptoms do not result from dopamine abnormalities. Recent studies have shown that these negative symptoms can be lessened by drugs that act on another neurotransmitter, gamma aminobutyric acid. Given the variable symptomatology of schizophrenia and the complexity of the brain systems involved, it is not surprising that continued progress is accompanied by new questions regarding the role of dopamine in this disease. Nevertheless, investigations into the neu-

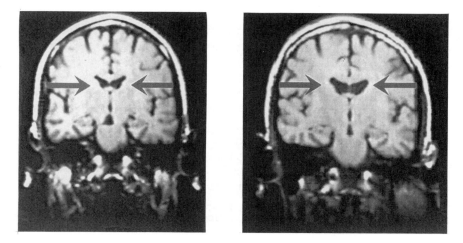

FIGURE 2-1 Magnetic resonance images of the brains of two 44-year-old male identical twins, one with schizophrenia (right) and the other without (left). Arrows point to the cerebral ventricles, which are enlarged in the affected twin. Images provided by the National Institute of Mental Health.

rochemical perturbations of schizophrenia have far-reaching implications for improved treatment of the disease. Digital maps of neurochemical systems, including the locations of different receptor subtypes, and the known functions of those systems in normal and disease states would be of particular value in the study of schizophrenia.

The ability to "image" the structure and functioning of the brain is a fundamental advance that is being vigorously applied to the study of schizophrenia. Magnetic resonance imaging (MRI) has revealed some subtle and intriguing structural abnormalities. These include in some individuals abnormally large cerebral ventricles, specific spaces in the brain containing cerebrospinal fluid, and an apparent thinning of certain areas of the cortex that are involved in emotional expression (Figure 2-1). Nevertheless, the functional implications of these structural abnormalities have yet to be determined. Brain imaging techniques, such as positron emission tomography (PET scanning) and its variations, can be used to measure such functions as energy metabolism, blood flow, and receptor binding; localized electrical activity can be recorded using electroencephalography and magnetoencephalography. These imaging studies can be done while subjects are actively involved in specific tasks or at rest. Such studies can also shed light on brain functioning during periods of severe dysfunction or relative remission, and during treatment with antischizophrenic medications. Studies of regional cerebral blood flow suggest decreased activation of the frontal cortex in response to certain tasks in some people with schizophrenia. PET studies of cerebral metabolism have confirmed this dampened activity of the frontal cortex and have further suggested increased activation of other brain regions. PET studies of dopamine receptor binding in schizophrenic patients are just beginning to yield interesting, although sometimes conflicting, information.

The potential of functional imaging studies to increase our knowledge of schizophrenia is great, but these studies are complicated by several factors. For example, the variable clusters of symptoms exhibited by different patients and their differing treatment histories must be carefully correlated with the specific findings from imaging experiments. In pharmacological studies, such as those that examine dopamine receptor binding, the differing properties of the drugs that are used must be well understood to interpret the results of each experiment. Databases of imaging data combined with careful annotations regarding patient history, pharmacological properties, and other variables could greatly facilitate more rapid and more meaningful conclusions from these types of studies.

Genetic studies, involving both population and molecular genetics, are integral to research on schizophrenia. Studies of families and particularly of twins clearly suggest genetic factors in the disease. Yet attempts to locate the "schizophrenia gene" have not been successful. Candidates include genes coding for the dopamine (D_2) receptor or for certain enzymes involved in dopamine synthesis or degradation. The lack of success in finding a likely single gene, combined with the complicated manifestations of the disease and the different responses to treatment, suggests that schizophrenia might actually be a group of related diseases. Indeed, strong evidence supports the notion that there is probably more than one gene related to schizophrenia and that instead of being a direct cause, it confers increased susceptibility for the disease.

This increased susceptibility raises the issue of environmental factors that might precipitate expression of such a genetic predisposition. Proposed factors range from viruses, or other infectious agents, to nutritional deficits to traumatic early childhood experiences. Information about these environmental factors and the varied clinical manifestations of the disease is exceedingly difficult to correlate. Therefore, another use for sophisticated information management tools is to begin to build a knowledge base about all that is known regarding the environmental history of each patient, in context with information about the pattern and prevalence of schizophrenia in their families. In addition, once candidate genes for increased susceptibility are identified, they can be compared with the genetic maps in existing databases (see Chapter 4).

Schizophrenia stands as yet another example of the brain's complexity. Better answers about the causes of and effective treatments for schizophrenia are anxiously awaited by those who suffer from the disease and by their families. Although more data are needed to provide these answers, there is also a pressing need to correlate and combine more adequately the data that already exist.

The Growth of Neuroscience

Neuroscience research has grown in response to critical problems

The costs of caring for those who suffer from neurological disorders, drug abuse, and mental illness, combined with the cost of lost wages and other indirect losses from these conditions, are extremely difficult to estimate because reporting mechanisms cannot account for those who have more than one disorder (e.g., hearing loss and Parkinson's disease) and the severity of these disorders vary widely. Yet even without such estimates we know that these disorders constitute a sizable liability to the health and well-being of U.S. society (Table 2-1). Nearly 23 million Americans suffer from neurological and communicative disorders resulting from head and spinal cord injury, hearing and speech impairments, and infectious diseases of the nervous system, including acquired immune deficiency syndrome (AIDS). More than 3.5 million people suffer the effects of debilitating disorders such as Alzheimer's, Parkinson's and Huntington's diseases, and demyelinating and atrophic disorders such as multiple sclerosis and amyotrophic lateral sclerosis (National Advisory Neurological and Communicative Disorders and Stroke Council, 1989; National Institute of Neurological Disorders and Stroke, 1989). Impairment arising from alcohol abuse, drug abuse, and mental illness also takes a significant toll. It is estimated that more than 60 million Americans suffer from such mental illnesses as schizophrenia, affective disorders, anxiety disorders, various types of dementia, eating disorders, childhood and adolescent disorders, and sleep disorders, and more than 20 million Americans suffer from alcohol or drug abuse (Alcohol, Drug Abuse, and Mental Health Administration, 1990; Gerstein and Harwood, 1990; Rice et al., 1990).

Researchers have estimated the lifetime prevalence for any alcohol, drug, or mental health (ADM) disorder to be 32.7 percent (Regier et al., 1990). Moreover, there is significant comorbidity among ADM

TABLE 2-1   Prevalence of Selected Neurological Disorders, Mental
Illnesses, and Alcohol and Drug Abuse

Condition	Estimated Cases (in millions)[a]
Alzheimer's disease and related dementias	3.0
Brain tumors	0.062
Epilepsy	2.0
Multiple sclerosis	0.131
Neuro-AIDS	0.02[b]
Stroke	1.9
Trauma (head and spinal cord injury)	1.0
Mental illnesses	
Affective disorders	27.7
Antisocial personality	8.8
Anxiety disorders	25.3
Schizophrenic disorders	2.6
Alcohol and drug abuse	
Alcohol	17.7
Drug	4.6
Total	94.8

[a]Some persons have more than one disorder concurrently (e.g., epilepsy and affective disorder), and these figures may reflect that comorbidity.
[b]Incidence (number of new cases reported each year).
SOURCE: For neurological disorders, NINDS, November 1989 and NANCDSC, January 1989; for mental illnesses, Rice et al., 1990; for alcohol and drug abuse, ADAMHA, 1990 and Gerstein and Harwood, 1990.

disorders. For example, the Regier study also showed that 37 percent of those with an alcohol disorder had a comorbid mental disorder; of patients with a drug disorder (other than alcohol), more than half (53 percent) had a mental disorder as well. The frontline efforts now occurring to understand and treat this diverse array of diseases are headed by basic and clinical neuroscientists.

Neuroscience has grown in response to new technologies and an expanded understanding of biology

Much of the recent growth in neuroscience has been spurred by the development of important enabling technologies, which have opened entirely new areas of research. For example, the development of the oscilloscope permitted the first accurate visualization of the electrical activity of neurons. The development of the electron microscope allowed investigators to study components of neurons too small to be seen with conventional microscopes. The development of antibody techniques to tag specific molecules permitted the visualization and localization of specific neurochemicals. In addition, the combination of tissue culture techniques with antibody labeling and molecular biological techniques has provided critical new knowledge regarding the mechanisms of neural functioning. Finally, the development of computer technologies has played a fundamental role over the past two decades in enabling data collection and analysis of single-neuron physiological data. More recently, the development of graphic visualization techniques has permitted researchers to view the active functioning of a human brain.

Many other factors in addition to technology have contributed to the growth of neuroscience—for example, increased appreciation of the importance of the fundamental biological processes that underlie brain disorders, especially mental illness. In the past decade, the groundwork has been laid for tackling some of the most intractable neurological problems, including spinal cord injury, epilepsy, stroke, and neurodegenerative diseases. These and other achievements have led to a feast of exciting research opportunities that have attracted great numbers of new investigators to neuroscience in the past 10 years. The Society for Neuroscience membership roster currently stands at more than 17,500, a remarkable figure, given that there were only 500 charter members in 1969 and 6,350 members in 1979. (At the society's annual meeting in 1990, almost 8,000 abstracts of individual research projects were presented.) Beyond U.S. borders, growth in international organizations is also apparent: the International Brain Research Organization boasts more than 20,000 members from 73 countries. An increase in scientific journals has accompanied this growth, with more than 200 scientific journals now exclusively devoted to neuroscience disciplines in the areas of basic science or clinical investigation.

Although growth in the field of neuroscience has contributed greatly to an understanding of the brain, it is not without its problems. The volume of knowledge and information generated from this work has been growing linearly with public and private investments in resources and with individual commitment. This expanding knowledge offers extraordinary opportunities for neuroscience to make rapid progress in the treatment and prevention of mental and neurological illnesses during the next decade. Without innovative strategies for information management, communication, and processing, however, the amount and complexity of the data present daunting impediments to future advances.

Neuroscience research is a national priority

A comprehensive resource for managing information on brain structure and functioning is necessary to protect an already substantial public investment. One measure of the current national investment in neuroscience research is federal and nonfederal expenditures. Tables 2-2a and 2-2b summarize the neuroscience-related expenditures of two agencies, the National Institutes of Health (NIH) and the Alcohol, Drug Abuse, and Mental Health Administration (ADAMHA). Many other agencies in the federal biomedical research complex also support basic, as well as clinical, neuroscience research. The National Science Foundation has a long history of funding basic neuroscience research, and other federal research support derives from such agencies as the Department of Energy, the Department of Veterans Affairs, and the Office of Naval Research (Table 2-3). Outside the federal government, a number of private agencies and foundations, such as the Howard Hughes Medical Institute and the MacArthur Foundation, provide support for neuroscience research (Table 2-3). Although it is impossible to determine the precise amount spent on neuroscience research (because of the diversity of funding sources and the inclusion of neuroscience-targeted funds in budgets that reflect support in more than one field of biomedical research), it is estimated that the total national investment is approximately $1.5 billion per year (Table 2-3).

When considered within the context of the massive disease burden from mental and neurological diseases, even greater investment in neuroscience research could be justified. Strategies such as the Brain Mapping Initiative are designed in part to protect current investments by maximizing the integration of information gained from neuroscience research. The long-term benefits of this research are numerous and will substantially reduce the national and international burden—both in terms of costs and human suffering—imposed by neurological and mental disorders. To hasten this progress, strategies must be developed to integrate new discoveries with the extensive body of accumulated knowledge. Such integration is needed now because the advances made by neuroscientists, especially in the past decade, have brought this research enterprise to the threshold of major breakthroughs in a number of areas, including neurogenetics, biobehavioral sciences, and neural injury. Neuroscience research is a complex field that comprises many subdisciplines, most of which share a common need for a comprehensive map of the brain in digital

TABLE 2-2a   Investment in Neuroscience Research (in thousands of dollars) by the National Institutes of Health

Institute	1988 (Actual)	1989 (Actual)	1990 (Estimated)
Division of Research Resources	30,301	34,365	28,728
National Cancer Institute	34,068	41,378	42,753
National Eye Institute	79,188	81,244	81,753
National Heart, Lung, and Blood Institute	52,970	56,280	57,700
National Institute of Allergy and Infectious Diseases	24,571	40,197	41,805
National Institute of Arthritis and Musculoskeletal and Skin Diseases	628	1,137	1,255
National Institute of Child Health and Human Development	78,173	91,032	95,000
National Institute of Dental Research	9,337	8,511	8,755
National Institute of Diabetes and Digestive and Kidney Diseases	25,500	26,900	28,100
National Institute of Environmental Health Sciences	15,588	19,120	19,866
National Institute of General Medical Sciences	11,400	11,500	11,750
National Institute of Neurological Disorders and Stroke	458,792	471,632	490,409
National Institute on Aging	63,221	78,573	84,380
Total	883,707	961,869	992,254

SOURCE: Division of Financial Management, National Institutes of Health, September 1990.

TABLE 2-2b   Investment in Neuroscience Research (in thousands of dollars) by the Alcohol, Drug Abuse, and Mental Health Administration[a]

Agency	1988	1989	1990
National Institute of Mental Health	118,803	153,881	180,161
National Institute on Drug Abuse	38,000	54,000	66,000
National Institute on Alcohol Abuse and Alcoholism	18,609	23,904	29,313
Total	175,412	231,785	275,474

[a]All numbers are actual.
SOURCE: Financial management and planning offices of the three agencies, December 1990.

TABLE 2-3 U.S. Investment (in thousands of dollars) in Neuroscience and Mental Health Research: Sponsoring Agencies and Foundations[a]

Unit	Amount[b]
National Institutes of Health	992,254
Alcohol, Drug Abuse, and Mental Health Administration	275,474
Department of Veterans Affairs	115,369[c]
National Science Foundation	39,000
Office of Naval Research	22,200
Department of Energy	20,000
Office of Scientific Research U.S. Air Force	15,600
Environmental Protection Agency	3,900[d]
Department of Agriculture	3,501
Centers for Disease Control	1,204[e]
Foundations	
Howard Hughes Medical Institute	35,000
The John D. and Catherine T. MacArthur Foundation	14,000
Pew Charitable Trusts	6,500[c]
Whitehall Foundation, Inc.	2,000
Total	1,546,002

[a]Includes basic and clinical, extramural and intramural research only (services excluded).

[b]Figures are for fiscal year 1990 except where otherwise indicated and were obtained through personal communications and, in some cases, annual reports.

[c]Fiscal year 1989 figures.

[d]Figure is for the Neurotoxicology Division of the Health Effects Research Laboratory.

[e]Extramural grants for head injury research.

form. The incorporation, through a Brain Mapping Initiative, of enabling technologies in the field of neuroscience research is an appropriate strategy to future breakthroughs.

References

Alcohol, Drug Abuse, and Mental Health Administration. 1990. Alcohol and Health (Seventh Special Report to the U.S. Congress). ADAMHA Pub. No. 90-1656. Washington, D.C.: U.S. Department of Health and Human Services, Public Health Service.

Barker, D., E. Wright, K. Nguyen, L. Cannon, P. Fain, D. Goldgar, D. T. Bishop, J. Carey, B. Baty, J. Kivlin, H. Willard, J. S. Waye, G. Greig, L. Leinwand, Y. Nakamura. P. O'Connell, M. Leppert, J.-M. Lalouel, R. White, and M. Skolnick. 1987. Gene for von Recklinghausen neurofibromatosis is in the pericentromeric region of chromosome 17. Science 236:1100–1102.

Colwell, R. R., ed. 1989. Biomolecular Data: A Resource in Transition. New York: Oxford University Press.

DeLisi, C. 1988. Computers in molecular biology: Current applications and emerging trends. Science 240:47–52.

Gerstein, D. R., and H. J. Harwood, eds. 1990. Treating Drug Problems, vol. 1. Washington, D.C.: National Academy Press.

Howard Hughes Medical Institute. 1990. Finding the Critical Shapes. Bethesda, Md.: Howard Hughes Medical Institute Office of Communications.

Hubel, D. H., and T. N. Wiesel. 1979. Brain mechanisms of vision. Scientific American 241(3):150–162.

Lewis, R. 1990. A glimpse of neurofibromatosis 1 protein function. Journal of NIH Research 2(Oct.):60–64.

McCormick, B. H., T. A. DeFanti, and M. D. Brown, eds. 1987. Visualization in scientific computing. SIGGRAPH Computer Graphics Newsletter 21(6):1–13.

National Advisory Neurological and Communicative Disorders and Stroke Council. 1989. Decade of the Brain: Answers Through Scientific Research. NIH Pub. No. 88-2957. Bethesda, Md.: U.S. Department of Health and Human Services, National Institutes of Health.

National Institute of Neurological Disorders and Stroke. 1989. Profile. Bethesda, Md.: U.S. Department of Health and Human Services, National Institutes of Health.

Regier, D. A., M. E. Farmer, D. S. Rae, B. Z. Locke, S. J. Keith, L. L. Judd, and F. K. Goodwin. 1990. Comorbidity of mental disorders with alcohol and other substance abuse. Journal of the American Medical Association 264(19):2511–2518.

Rice, D. P., S. Kelman, L. S. Miller, and S. Dunmeyer, eds. 1990. The Economic Costs of Alcohol and Drug Abuse and Mental Illness. ADAMHA Pub. No. 90-1694. Washington, D.C.: U.S. Department of Health and Human Services, Alcohol, Drug Abuse, and Mental Health Administration.

Rowbotham, M. C., and H. L. Fields. 1989. Post-herpetic neuralgia: The relation of pain complaint, sensory disturbance, and skin temperature. Pain 39:129–144.

Sacks, O. 1970. The Man Who Mistook His Wife for a Hat. New York: Harper and Row.

Seizinger, B. R., G. A. Rouleau, L. J. Ozelius, A. H. Lane, A. G. Faryniarz, M. V. Chao, S. Huson, B. R. Korf, D. M. Parry, M. A. Pericak-Vance, and J. Gusella. 1987. Genetic linkage of von Recklinghausen neurofibromatosis to the nerve growth factor receptor gene. Cell 49(5):589–594.

Smith, T. F. 1990. The history of the genetic sequence databases. Genomics 6:701-707.

Vela, C. 1990. Overview of U.S. Genome and Selected Scientific Databases. Background paper prepared for the Committee on a National Neural Circuitry Database, Institute of Medicine.

3

Overview of Neuroscience Research: A Closer Look at the Neural Hierarchy

This chapter is intended as a primer or simplified overview of some aspects of neuroscience for those readers not familiar with the field. As such, the chapter describes some of the experiments that are done at each level of a vertical hierarchy of neural functioning, from behavior to genetic mechanisms (Figure 3-1). Researchers have developed hundreds of techniques and formulated elaborate repertoires of experimental strategies to answer fundamental questions about brain functions. When combined, these techniques provide information at all levels of the vertical hierarchy. Although apparently distinct, these levels cannot be separated because information that exists at one horizontal plane must be considered in concert with information from all other planes to generate a coherent picture of brain functioning. In addition, at each vertical level, the results of many different experimental approaches need to be integrated.

Behavior and emotion are manifestations of brain activity

Behavior encompasses many degrees of complexity, from the most rudimentary knee-jerk reflex to the subtlety and sophistication of movement exhibited by a ballet dancer or chess grand master. The study of behavior can be subdivided into several broad facets: sensory processing (vision, hearing, touch, and smell leading to conscious perception), motor processing (reflexes and coordinated movements), and cognitive processing (learning, thinking, and planning). Behavior also includes psychological processes, such as personality and mood.

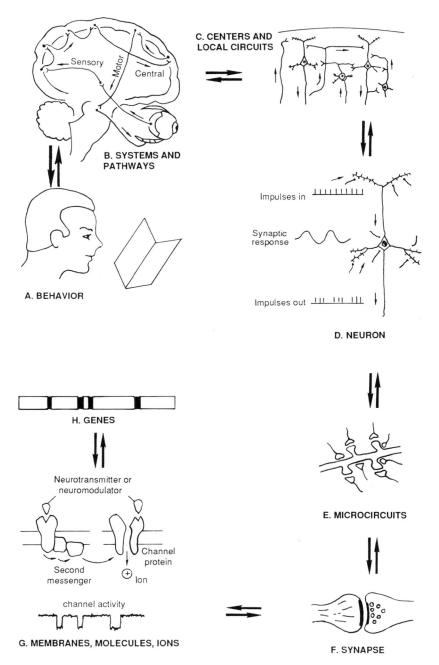

FIGURE 3-1 The neural hierarchy. Adapted from Shepherd, 1988.

Animals as simple as fruit flies and snails exhibit behaviors that are neurally driven. As organisms become more complex, their behaviors become correspondingly more intricate. Human behavior represents the ultimate in rich and elaborate repertoires that are affected by a range of factors from "hard-wired" genetic codes to minute-by-minute environmental perturbations. Behavior and its neural underpinnings must also be understood across different developmental stages and different abnormal or pathological conditions. The challenge in neuroscience is to understand the contributions of different factors to specific behavioral and emotional functions. Because important factors exist at all levels of the hierarchy, from organized brain systems to individual cells and even genes, this formidable challenge can be met only by invoking a diverse and powerful arsenal of experimental tools.

Many behavioral studies in animals employ conditioning techniques first developed by Pavlov in the late 1920s. By pairing a bell with the presentation of food to a dog, Pavlov was able to "condition" the dog to respond physiologically with increased gastric secretion when only the bell was sounded and no food was present. (In other words, a bell/food association was established, and this mental association produced a physiological response in the animal's body.) Later research efforts developed the concept of operant conditioning: animals can be taught, using associations of food and sensory stimuli such as sound or light, to press bars, enter doors, or perform some other activity. Moreover, once an animal is trained to perform a specific activity, new associations can be taught; how well these activities are learned, as well as the disruption of well-learned activities, can then be assessed using a variety of experimental manipulations. For example, many psychotropic drugs, including morphine and nicotine, have been tested by operant conditioning in studies aimed at finding replacement drugs that are perceived by the user to be similar to the real drug but that have no addictive properties. Finally, because operant conditioning models involve learning, behavioral experiments with rats born of alcohol-ingesting mothers or rats exposed to lead poisoning have contributed to an understanding of some of the learning deficits that result from prenatal or environmental exposure to toxic substances.

Other behavioral research has involved the selective destruction or electrical stimulation of discrete brain regions and the subsequent observation of behavioral changes. Such experiments helped to associate a particular part of the hypothalamus with the regulation of eating behavior, certain limbic system nuclei with aggressive behavior, specific nuclei of the diencephalon with a variety of movement disorders, and the hippocampus with memory deficits. As more is learned about the presence, function, and location of brain neurotransmitters and neuromodulators, these kinds of investigations are expanding to measure the effects of loss and replacement of specific neurochemicals.

Learning and memory can also be measured in nonhuman animals. Simple organisms, such as the fruit fly, can be classically conditioned, and, amazingly, certain specific genetic mutations in the fruit fly are known to compromise severely this type of learning (Dudai, 1985). Because there are important similarities, or homologies, between the genes of fruit flies and those of higher animals, identification of the protein encoded by the defective gene may provide a clue to the genetic basis of learning in higher animals.

Animals such as monkeys are capable of complex learning tasks— for example, long chains of discrete movements, association of symbols with specific movements, association between different objects, or manipulation of spatial relationships between objects. These tasks can be designed in such a way as to distinguish short-term memory from long-term memory and to allow precise measurement of learning acquisition. Behaviors such as these can then be used as benchmarks for a range of manipulations of brain structure and chemistry. Electrical recordings of brain activity made during specific tasks can help localize the part of the brain that mediates the information processing and control of movements necessary for the task. These tasks are also useful for assessing the deficits caused by experimental brain injury or stroke.

The aim of behavioral research in animals is to discover neural processes that can be correlated with human brain functions. Yet the techniques applied to human behavior have also sought to go beyond such correlations and acquire a window into cognitive and emotional function. For a long time, behavioral research in humans was severely limited by the paucity of techniques appropriate for human experimentation. Now, a number of new techniques permit the study of human brain function. One important step was the advent of noninvasive recording methods such as electroencephalographic (EEG) recordings, which made it possible to associate certain behavioral states with changes in the electrical activity of the cerebral cortex. (The recordings exhibit different patterns during different states of consciousness, including quiet wakefulness, alert wakefulness, and sleep.) Following its development, the EEG technique was immediately applied to the study of many human neurological and mental illnesses.

More recently, it has become possible to discriminate between different kinds of brain electrical activity by amplifying particular components of the EEG recordings during stimulation of specific visual, auditory, or sensory systems. These so-called event-related potential (ERP) recordings, which are essentially more finely tuned EEGs, contain specific waveforms that can be mapped, albeit with limited resolution, to specific structures of the brain. ERPs have been used to diagnose brain injury locations, describe abnormalities in schizophrenic patients, and trace the pathways underlying certain types of information processing. In the past five years, techniques have begun to be developed to record the magnetic rather than electrical fields that are generated by cortical activity. Magnetoencephalography, or neuromagnetic imaging, has been applied to the study of epileptic seizure activity and may in the future add greater resolution to the study of human brain activity.

Another exciting development is the ability to measure simultaneously the activity of most of the discrete brain regions in humans, during a variety of situations, with positron emission tomography. In PET scanning, short-lived radioactive markers are attached to specific molecules and injected into the bloodstream. These tagged molecules can then be visualized by detectors outside the brain and the resulting images stored in a computer (Plate 3-1). In some cases, the tagged molecules trace the blood flow to or the uptake of glucose by the brain. Tracing these patterns in the nervous system helps to identify brain regions with higher activity levels—they generally exhibit increased blood flow and increased uptake of glucose. Likewise, decreased blood flow and glucose uptake are associated with those brain regions that are not as active or that are being inhibited. Researchers have also used PET to visualize the binding of various drugs and neurotransmitter substances to receptors in the brain during discrete behavioral tasks and in certain emotional states.

Because PET studies can be repeated several times, they can be used to evaluate clinical treatments for behavioral and emotional disorders, in addition to their use in diagnosis or basic research. PET screening permits the reassessment of individual subjects after the administration of therapeutic agents or therapies and thus may show a return to or approximation of normal brain activity following successful therapies. Clearly, the use of PET in normal subjects also has great potential for increasing basic understanding of the brain and its processes in addition to providing a baseline from which to judge experimental therapies. So far, PET has provided the best and most complete information on humans with which to correlate the mass of data from studies of nonhuman animals, and its use will facilitate a more rapid transfer of basic science research to human beings.

Magnetic resonance imaging is another technology that has proved to be useful in visualizing brain functions. MRI uses external magnetic fields to visualize the three-dimensional structure of the brain at a resolution much better than that provided by x-rays or computer-assisted tomography (CT). Even though MR and CT images are essentially views of static structures and do not reflect dynamic changes, their improved resolution has had an immediate impact on the localization of brain damage from stroke, Alzheimer's disease, epilepsy, and brain cancer. Furthermore, numerous efforts are under way to achieve the precise overlay, or registration, of MR images with PET images so that the anatomical localization of PET data can be improved. The future should see the improvement of MRI techniques to allow visualization of particular molecules, such as phosphorus, to reveal dynamic changes in neurochemical activity over time.

The systems of the brain are connected by elaborate pathways and serve many functions

Although behavioral research has associated many functions with specific parts of the brain, resolution of precisely how neural computation occurs depends on knowledge of how various brain regions are connected to each other and how activity in one region affects other regions. This level of the hierarchy is concerned with organized groups of neurons—"areas" of the cerebral cortex and "nuclei" of subcortical regions. Groups of nuclei and areas make up the major systems of the brain, and vast networks of connections link these components. At the turn of the century, the development and use of histochemical stains revealed the rich variety of neuronal types and allowed researchers to map and identify many of the interconnections among major systems of the brain.

For many years this early information guided initial studies of factors crucial to the development of certain brain regions. For example, research showed that the neurons in the visual part of the cerebral cortex in kittens, who were prevented from seeing by birth defects or experimental closing of the eyelids at birth, did not develop properly. This finding provided the important knowledge that proper development depended on the ability of the system to function (also see Box 2-2).

More recent developments include neuroanatomical tract tracing techniques to analyze the circuitry of the brain. These techniques take advantage of the fact that neurons absorb certain substances, which subsequently move from the axonal endings to the cell body or from the cell body to the axonal endings. These tracer substances can be made visible in a number of ways, and their presence or absence in specific regions of the brain indicates whether a region has connections to some other region. In other words, the substances allow investigators to demonstrate a connection between the region of the brain in which the substance was placed and the region to which it was transported. Sometimes it is possible to visualize the tracers, through high magnification with an electron microscope, in axonal endings that contact one specific neuron. Such high-resolution studies have determined that these connections are often to a specific part of a neuron and occur in a highly predictable pattern. In addition, by using more than one of these tracing substances at a time, it is possible to map multiple pathways of connections among neurons and neuron groups. Complementing the anatomical research have been electrophysiological studies of brain pathways and systems. Such efforts not only establish circuitry information but often shed light on the functional relationships between certain regions (because physiological responses to stimulation, such as excitation and inhibition, can also be measured).

Much of the present understanding of the networks of the brain has come from anatomical and physiological studies such as those described above. This work has generated conceptual frameworks that have greatly advanced our thinking about the brain and that have been borrowed by computer scientists who are attempting to build "thinking" computers. A key framework from these studies is the concept of parallel distributed processing of information. Rarely is there just one brain pathway for a certain type of information; instead, many pathways, involving tens of millions of neurons, run parallel to each other. Nevertheless, information is selectively distributed to specific regions of the brain by functionally distinct processing streams. This organization underlies the brain's ability to store, process, and mediate hundreds of kinds of information simultaneously and reliably.

Overlying the anatomically defined neural systems are the chemical systems of the brain. It is common for particular neurotransmitter substances to predominate in specific brain nuclei, and thus knowledge about the actions of these neurotransmitter substances must be added to knowledge of the known anatomical connections of a particular brain region. The functional importance of the interaction of anatomical and chemical systems is particularly well illustrated in a region of the brain known as the substantia nigra. This region contains many neurons that contain the neurotransmitter dopamine, and the loss of these neurons is responsible for most of the effects noted in Parkinson's disease (Plate 3-2).

Techniques for defining these chemical systems began to be developed in biochemical studies, which isolated bioactive neurochemicals from specific brain regions. As these neurochemicals were character- ized, their effects in discrete nuclei were assessed by a variety of techniques—for example, injecting tiny amounts of the neurochemi- cal into the brain and recording the physiological response, or inject- ing the substance and measuring changes in an animal's behavior. A major breakthrough in the study of neurochemical systems was the development of antibody labeling techniques, or immunocytochem- istry, in which antibodies are obtained that recognize and bind to a specific neurochemical. The antibodies can be tagged in various ways and used to visualize the neurochemical's specific locations in the brain. Very soon after this discovery, researchers had developed spe- cific antibodies that recognized a number of neurochemicals (or their synthetic enzymes), and detailed maps of the locations of these neu- rotransmitters in the brain began to emerge. Throughout the past 10 years, detailed maps of the locations of scores of neurotransmitters and neuromodulators have been generated. Furthermore, techniques have been developed that combine tract tracing methods with im- munocytochemistry and thus reveal simultaneously the connections and neurochemistry of discrete brain regions. Finally, the changes in these maps during development and following injury have been and continue to be actively examined.

Neurons come in many shapes and sizes, and contain different chemicals

Neurons are the signaling cells or basic functional units of the brain (Box 3-1). Each neuron has three major parts: cell body, den- drites, and axon. The cell body is the neuron's powerhouse and contains the biosynthetic machinery for making proteins and other molecules needed by the cell. Extensions of the cell body (processes), called dendrites, normally form a multitude of branching patterns, accounting in part for the many different shapes neurons exhibit. Most of the surface area of neurons is in the dendrites, which are the primary receivirg areas for signals from other neurons. Neurons have only one axon extending from their cell bodies; the axon trans- mits neural signals from the cell body to other cells. All neurons are electrically charged (like a battery) as a result of different ion con- centrations inside and outside the cell. When a neuron is excited, ions flow through the cell's membrane, and the voltage difference between inside and outside is briefly reversed. This voltage reversal, called an action potential, is propagated down the axon to its end- ings, where it causes the release of the neurotransmitters stored with- in these endings.

Many different kinds of neurochemicals are transported back and

BOX 3-1 NOT ALL NEUROSCIENCE RESEARCH IS CONCERNED WITH NEURONS

Glia are the supporting cells of the brain and are not involved in synaptic transmission. More numerous than neurons, glial cells perform a variety of functions. For example, they constitute the insulating myelin sheaths that cover many axons. Microglia ingest debris from brain injury or normal cell death. Another type of glial cell guides the migration of developing neurons. Following brain injuries, glia proliferate and form scars. As researchers develop new methods to encourage injured axons to regrow, such scars could present a serious barrier.

The **blood-brain barrier** is a physical barrier between the blood and brain tissue, formed by special junctions between the cells lining the cerebral blood vessels. The brain is exquisitely sensitive to changes in acidity, extracellular protein content, and other factors. The blood-brain barrier protects the brain from these changes by preventing many chemicals from entering the brain's extracellular spaces. However, the barrier also prevents many therapeutic agents, including anticancer and antibiotic drugs, from reaching the site of tumors or infections. Research has revealed some mechanisms for bypassing the blood-brain barrier and has identified conditions under which the barrier is disrupted.

forth to the cell body in axons, sometimes along specialized protein structures (microtubules) that are like railroads along which little packets (e.g., vesicles containing neurotransmitters) of material can travel. (These same packets are sometimes responsible for transporting the pathway-tracing substances mentioned in the previous section.) Axons are important in development because directed growth of the axon from the developing neuron to its intended targets is critical to proper development of a whole brain. Although such growth is affected by a host of chemical cues and mechanisms, the transport of certain "trophic" factors by the axon is a key aspect of the growth process.

In addition to the more than 100 major neuronal types defined by size and shape, neurons differ in the kind of neurotransmitters and neuromodulators they produce. More than a hundred of these neurochemicals have been identified, and the list continues to grow. Some act to excite or to inhibit other neurons, and some act in subtle ways to enhance or depress these effects. Investigation of the regional location of specific neurotransmitters has indicated a role for the neurotransmitter acetylcholine in Alzheimer's disease. Analysis with immunocytochemistry in many regions has further revealed that many neurons contain and release more than one neurochemical at a time. Moreover, the balance of functionally important neurochemicals may change during development. Sometimes one cell type can be the locus for significant neurological dysfunctions—as mentioned earlier, the specific population of cells that are damaged in Parkinson's disease. All of these factors must be studied to map the structural and functional organization of each region of the brain and spinal cord.

Researchers also employ electrophysiological techniques at the cellular level of analysis, which often involves the penetration of individual cells with microscopically small electrodes to study the activity of a single cell. A recently developed physiological technique that shows great promise is the use of voltage- and ion-sensitive dyes (Plate 3-3). These dyes are fluorescent substances that are taken up by neurons and that change colors depending on the voltage state of the cell or the ion content of the cytoplasm inside the neuron. Special microscopes can record these color changes (in response to a variety of experimental manipulations) and provide images of the changes over time and in discrete regions of the neuron. Researchers have applied this technique to the study of regional activation of specific neuronal types, activity of specific neurotransmitters, and activity of developing neurons.

Another recently developed technique, in situ hybridization, employs specially synthesized pieces of nucleic acids that have a sequence complementary to the RNA that codes for specific proteins within neurons. These complementary pieces, which can be tagged with radioactive labels, bind to the RNA of interest; exposing brain tissue to these probes, the presence and quantity of RNA coding for specific proteins can be visualized and measured (Plate 3-4). This technique is particularly valuable because it can measure, through the changes in RNA synthesis, the effect of many variables, including neural activity, on genetic regulation of protein synthesis.

Considerable overlap occurs between investigations at the cellular level, such as those described here, and investigations at the systems, synaptic, and molecular levels. In many respects, the individual cells are the nodal points where the various molecular and genetic processes combine to give rise to the structural and gross functional organization of the nervous system. Thus, investigators at many levels of the neural hierarchy must consider the information their efforts generate within the context of the neuronal types to which their data may apply.

Synapses and microcircuits filter vast numbers of messages

Synapses are highly specialized regions of neurons at which communication between cells takes place. Structurally, most synapses are polarized, in that the sending part of one neuron (an axonal ending) makes contact with the receiving part of another neuron (usually a cell body or dendrite). Between these two components is a small space, called the synaptic cleft. When an action potential occurs in the sending, or *pre*synaptic, neuron, it causes the release of neurotransmitter substances into the synaptic cleft. These substances diffuse across the space and bind to specific receptor molecules on the receiving, or *post*synaptic, neuron. Because each neuron is studded with literally thousands of synapses, any one synapse contributes only a tiny amount to excitation or inhibition of a cell. An action potential is produced if the excitatory inputs to the cell outweigh the inhibitory inputs (Figure 3-2). Underlying this process are complex biophysical mechanisms related to the properties of the neuronal membrane and to the precise location and distribution of different kinds of inputs.

The structural aspects of synapses and synapse formation are most often studied using an electron microscope. Such investigations have delineated many of the cellular specializations that occur at the synapse and have described the function of these specializations. One of the most interesting phenomena documented by electron microscopic studies is the retraction of presynaptic axonal endings, which results from various types of damage to the presynaptic cell. Such retraction can be transient or permanent and, depending on the number of lost synaptic inputs, can fundamentally change the balance of inputs to the postsynaptic cell. The loss of synapses may also cause structural changes in the postsynaptic cells, which are often visible in regular microscopic analysis. For example, in many large neurons of the cerebral cortex, dendrites have tiny projections called dendritic spines. The density of these spines, which provide even more surface area for synapses, has been shown to decrease with advanced age, an effect that can also occur in certain neurological disease states (Plate 3-5).

The physiology of synaptic transmission has been investigated using a variety of electrophysiological techniques in a wide range of animal species. These experiments, combined with chemical analysis, provide a rich picture of the many events that occur in the synaptic endings and in the postsynaptic neurons: ionic changes, the release of precise amounts of neurotransmitters, and actions, in the synaptic cleft, of enzymes that sometimes degrade neurotransmitters and thus end their effects. For example, researchers know that the amount of transmitter released depends on changes in the intracellular concentration of calcium in the axonal ending. This characteristic provides a mechanism by which synaptic transmission can be modified or reg-

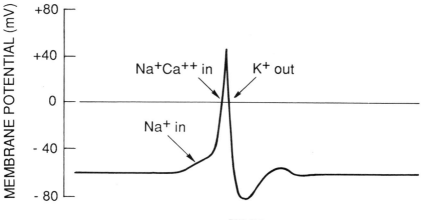

FIGURE 3-2 An action potential tracing. The action potential, the basis of neuronal signaling, is an electrical impulse generated by a change in the permeability of the cell membrane to sodium, calcium, potassium, and other ions. Adapted from Kandel and Schwartz, 1985.

ulated (varying the amount of transmitter that is released changes the likelihood of action potential generation in the postsynaptic cell). This ability to change is called plasticity and is another hallmark of neural information processing that computer scientists would like to reproduce in "thinking" computers.

Regulation of synaptic transmission has a number of interesting effects. It has been known for a long time that when a neuron is repeatedly stimulated, it often stops firing, despite continued stimulation. This process is known as habituation and is an adaptive response that helps filter out stimuli. Researchers have shown that repeated stimulation of a presynaptic ending results eventually in a decrease in the calcium entering the ending. The synapse then "loses its strength," so that presynaptic action potentials result in decreased release of neurotransmitter. A reverse mechanism, called sensitization, helps strengthen particular inputs.

By balancing inputs and filtering out unnecessary information, these mechanisms are probably critical to the microcircuitry involved in learning and memory. Many different brain regions are likely to be involved in various aspects of memory and learning, but a common theme for all of them is the strengthening of certain inputs over others on the cellular and synaptic levels. Many investigators in the field of computational neuroscience are concerned with defining the mathematical constraints of these processes. Their goal is to develop a deeper understanding of the nature of information storage in the brain and how it differs from information storage in conventional computers.

Messages can change molecular states and genetic expression

Neural signaling comprises much more than stimulus-response patterns. The molecular chemistry involved in transducing neural signals is an area of intense scientific interest and often serves as the point at which pharmacological treatments intervene. Excitation and inhibition of a neuron are mediated by ion channels that selectively regulate the flow of small ions, especially sodium, calcium, potassium, or chloride ions. Each ion channel is a complex molecule that is embedded in the cell membrane and contains a pore through which particular ions can pass. Most ion channels are either open or closed; these states are often "gated," or determined, by specific external influences. Some channels are gated by the action of neurotransmitters, others by the voltage difference across the membrane, and still others by mechanical stimuli, as occurs in peripheral nerve endings to signal touch and pressure on the skin. The regulation of gated channels gives rise to action potentials and involves many different types of biochemical reactions that have implications for all kinds of excitable membranes in the body, including skeletal and cardiac muscle cells, egg cells of the ovary, and certain immune system cells.

The first step in synaptic transmission is the binding of a neurotransmitter to a *receptor*—similar to a key in a lock. Some receptors actually form an ion channel when activated, and neurotransmitter binding to the receptor changes the structure of the pore so as to facilitate or inhibit ions from crossing the membrane. A specific type of acetylcholine receptor, which mediates muscle movement, is part of an ion channel, as are certain receptor subtypes for gamma aminobutyric acid (GABA), the receptor at which certain tranquilizers, such as Valium®, act. Other neurotransmitter-receptor complexes, however, initiate a complicated cascade of biochemical reactions that culminate in the structural modification of distinct ion channels. Such cascades involve so-called second messenger molecules, which function to activate other molecules.

Cyclic adenosine monophosphate (cAMP), a nucleotide molecule, is the best understood of these second messengers. cAMP is formed after many neurotransmitters attach to their receptors—including the type of receptor for norepinephrine that mediates increases in heart rate and is blocked by the beta blocker drugs that many heart patients take. At this receptor, the binding of transmitters causes the linking of the receptor to a protein, called a G protein, which transduces the signal by activating an enzyme (adenylate cyclase) that in turn causes the production of cAMP (Figure 3-3). cAMP then activates other enzymes (protein kinases) that cause phosphate groups to be added to other molecules, some of which may interact with the ion channel proteins. To make matters even more complex, some G proteins are inhibitory and some excitatory to this cascade. Other

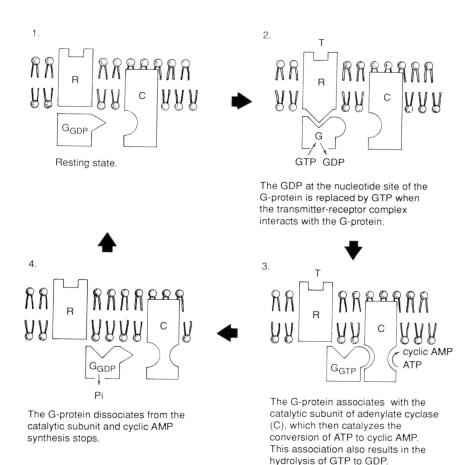

1.

Resting state.

2.

GTP GDP

The GDP at the nucleotide site of the G-protein is replaced by GTP when the transmitter-receptor complex interacts with the G-protein.

4.

Pi

The G-protein dissociates from the catalytic subunit and cyclic AMP synthesis stops.

3.

cyclic AMP
ATP

The G-protein associates with the catalytic subunit of adenylate cyclase (C), which then catalyzes the conversion of ATP to cyclic AMP. This association also results in the hydrolysis of GTP to GDP.

FIGURE 3-3 The synthesis of cyclic adenosine monophosphate (cAMP) that results when transmitter (T) binds to the beta-adrenergic receptor (R) is mediated through a transducer, or G-protein (G). GTP = guanosine triphosphate; GDP = guanosine diphosphate. Adapted from Kandel and Schwartz, 1985.

second messengers are lipids such as diacylglycerol, which activates protein kinase C in a cascade of chemical reactions usually distinct from that involving cAMP. Calcium, sometimes bound to proteins such as calmodulin, is yet a third second messenger that functions to activate a number of different enzymes. It is important to note that the chemical reaction cascades involving the three second messengers described here often intersect at key molecular points, allowing the different messenger systems to interact with each other.

Second messenger systems are a good example of the concept that the effects of synaptic transmission are not limited to the regulation of ion channels and the resulting excitation or inhibition of action potentials. Synaptic transmission also influences, to a greater or lesser degree, all of the biosynthetic processes of the cell, from the synthesis of neurotransmitters and receptors to the synthesis of proteins necessary to maintain the cell's structure. Such effects are the late consequences of cell activation and involve the regulation of genetic expression.

Certain genes found in human cells, including brain cells, are similar to viral genes implicated in cancer. These so-called proto-oncogenes have been found in brain cells, and it is thought that these genes function as third messengers because they code for proteins that in turn regulate gene expression. Soon after nerve injury, the expression of one of these oncogenes, called *cfos*, increases. The functional importance of this increase is not known but, among other possibilities, may well have important consequences for cellular repair. As mentioned previously, neurons synthesize different amounts of neurotransmitters and other neurochemicals depending on the developmental stage of the organism and other factors. The genetic regulation that controls the balance of these biosynthetic processes is another area with critical implications for normal and pathological brain functioning as well as for the response of the brain to injury.

Neuroscientists are also investigating the genes contained in cells of the nervous system through gene mapping, gene and protein sequencing techniques, and antibody techniques. For example, antibodies can be used to isolate a substance—a complex protein, for example—whose molecular structure is not known but whose presence is critical to some aspect of neural function. Once the molecular structure is known, it is then possible to find the gene that codes for that protein. Conversely, one can also use the genes as starting points to isolate and characterize a specific protein. Application of techniques that permit the isolation and sequencing of proteins has elucidated the structure of the acetylcholine receptor mentioned earlier (Figure 3-4). The receptor is composed of four large, related molecules (called sub-units, and one of these is repeated so that five molecules make

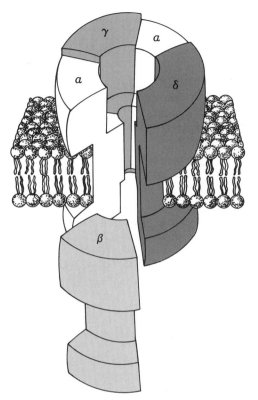

FIGURE 3-4 A three-dimensional model of the "spool-shaped" acetylcholine receptor. Adapted from Kandel and Schwartz, 1985.

up the receptor) that are arranged in a shape that resembles a thick spool. The center of the spool is open and provides a channel through which ions can pass. Each subunit of the receptor is coded by a separate messenger RNA (mRNA), which have now been sequenced, leading to a greater understanding of the structures of the genes themselves. Changes in gene expression, measured by assay of the mRNAs for each subunit, have shown that, in the developing junction between nerve and muscle, release of specific peptides from the growing axons causes activation of the acetylcholine receptor genes and stimulation of receptor synthesis. Such experimental strategies can now be applied to the study of the molecular and genetic effects of neurotransmitters, neuromodulators, and hormones that affect brain cells and, ultimately, behavior.

The application of molecular biological and genetic techniques in

BOX 3-2   THE GENETICS OF COLOR VISION

On the deepest surface of the retina lie the primary receptors of the human eye, called rods and cones. Rod cells, responsible for black-and-white vision in dim light, are far more numerous than cone cells, which enable us to perceive colors. Although Isaac Newton discovered the color spectrum some 300 years ago, it was not until the late eighteenth century that scientists began to understand the basis of color vision: light-absorbing proteins called pigments that have overlapping but distinct sensitivities to particular wavelengths of the visible spectrum. There are three classes of cone cells: those containing red pigment, those containing green pigment, and those containing blue.

Scientists now know that colorblindness, or the inablilty to discriminate red and green, results from alterations in the genes that encode these color pigments in the cone cells. That deficiencies in red-green discrimination are more common in males than in females is explained by the fact that the gene responsible for the variation is located in the X chromosome. Males will be colorblind if the single X chromosome they inherit from their mother carries the trait; females will be affected only if both their X chromosomes are variant. Aberrations in blue sensitivity, which affect males and females equally, are rooted in a gene on another, non-sex chromosome.

In hopes of supplementing the findings of these classic genetic studies, Jeremy Nathans and his colleagues at the Johns Hopkins University School of Medicine applied modern scientific techniques to the puzzle of abnormal color vision (Nathans, 1989). Using DNA hybridization, they isolated the genes that code for the color pigments of the cone cells and compared their structures in people with normal and variant color vision. Interestingly, they discovered that although people have only one copy of the gene that codes for red pigment, they have two or three copies of the gene that codes for green pigment. When multiple copies of a gene exist next to each other in this way, the copies have a tendency to recombine in peculiar patterns when cell division occurs, a phenomenon called unequal homologous recombination. Of the 25 subjects studied by Nathans with abnormal red-green discrimination, all but one had DNA that had been shuffled as a result of unequal homologous recombination, confirming the hypothesis that when green pigment genes rearrange themselves "unequally" or irregularly, deficiencies in color vision result.

Although much remains to be learned about the roles of cones and pigments in color vision, the work of Nathans and his colleagues yields interesting clues to the genetics behind what we see and what we cannot see.

neuroscience is very recent and quite promising. Recent landmark successes in neurogenetics have direct application to human health. As scientists identify and characterize ion channels, proteins, receptors, and neurotransmitters that play a role in disease, they gain clues to the location of the genes that control the production of these elements (Box 3-2). Already some neurological diseases are yielding to this approach. The genetic locus for Huntington's disease was discovered by an interdisciplinary group of researchers and has led to a test that predicts with remarkable accuracy whether a person at risk for Huntington's will develop the disease. The abnormal (mutated) genes for Duchenne's muscular dystrophy and neurofibromatosis have also been identified. In the case of muscular dystrophy, identification of the defective gene led to isolation of the protein dystrophin, for which the gene codes. Information about dystrophin may well permit scientists to design treatment strategies to replace the defective protein. Identification of the gene for neurofibromatosis is also beginning to lead researchers to important clues about the mechanism of that disease (see Box 2-1). Advances such as these are the necessary first steps in disease prevention, but further progress depends on basic scientific investigation into the regulation and expression of neural genes and the functional consequences of that expression in the brain.

References and Bibliography

Dudai, Y. 1985. Genes, enzymes, and learning in *Drosophila*. Trends in Neuroscience 8:18–21.

German, D. C., K. Manaye, W. K. Smith, D. J. Woodward, and C. B. Saper. 1989. Midbrain dopaminergic cell loss in Parkinson's disease: Computer visualization. Annals of Neurology 26:507–514.

Kandel, E. R., and J. H. Schwartz, eds. 1985. Principles of Neural Science. New York: Elsevier.

Nathans, J. 1989. The genes for color vision. Scientific American 260(2):42–49.

Pavlov, I. P. 1927. Conditioned Reflexes: An Investigation of the Physiological Activity of the Cerebral Cortex, G. V. Anrep, trans. London: Oxford University Press.

Shepherd, G. M. 1988. Neurobiology, 2nd ed. New York: Oxford University Press.

Tank, D. W., M. Sugimori, J. A. Connor, and R. R. Llinas. 1988. Spatially resolved calcium dynamics of mammalian purkinje cells in cerebellar slice. Science 242:773–777.

The following sources were also used as background for preparation of this chapter but are not cited specifically in the text.

Darnell, J., H. Lodish, and D. Baltimore. 1986. Molecular Cell Biology. New York: Scientific American Books, Inc.

Kelner, K. L., and D. E. Koshland, eds. 1989. Molecules to Models: Advances in Neuroscience. Papers from Science 1986–1989. AAAS Pub. No. 89-17S. Washington, D.C.: American Association for the Advancement of Science.

Kuffler, S. W., and J. G. Nichols. 1977. From Neuron to Brain: A Cellular Approach to the Function of the Nervous System. Sunderland, Mass.: Sinauer Assoc., Inc.

Ottoson, D., and W. Rostène, eds. 1989. Visualization of Brain Functions. New York: Stockton Press.

4
Computer and Information Technology in Biomedical and Neuroscience Research

A complex of computer-based resources that can greatly enhance neuroscience research is an attainable goal. Current trends in information technology offer an unprecedented opportunity for neuroscientists to expand their use of hard-won data and to communicate these data more effectively to other scientists. In addition, the sheer mass of neuroscience information accumulated to date and the accelerating rate at which new results are being obtained and reported are becoming major driving forces for the kind of organization, structure, and accessibility that computer-based resources can provide. The attractiveness of the present opportunity is also strengthened by the increasingly intimate role of various computer-based instruments and applications in neuroscience research. This chapter describes how a complex of electronic and digital resources for neuroscience might work in the future, and supports this description with examples obtained in part from the task forces organized to provide advice to the committee and the open hearings the committee sponsored. The chapter also dis-cusses the increasing reliance of biomedical research on computerized resources and the current trends in computer science and information technology that make the goal of a complex of resources attainable.

A neuroscience laboratory of the future will use a variety of computer-based tools

The neuroscience laboratory of the future may seem incredible from our present viewpoint. But a neuroscientist who had fallen asleep over the microscope in 1970 would awaken today to an equally incredible vision of color graphics workstations, shiny compact disks containing masses of data, and electronic mail messages from colleagues worldwide. Any projections of the future we might generate today are likely to fall short, in some respects, of what will be possible by 2010.

The following scenario illustrates how an experiment might be done in a neuroscience laboratory of the future. (The physiological, anatomical, and biochemical processes it describes are consistent with known aspects of neural function.) Although it is hypothetical and overly simplified, it makes explicit the vision of a family of inter-related databases and other computer-based resources for neuroscience research. Further, it illustrates how three-dimensional graphics, databases, networks, and electronic journals will contribute to research that proceeds more rapidly and efficiently than anything we can imagine today, transcending present conventional information boundaries.

The futuristic scene opens in the laboratory of Jane Smith, who is studying a brain region recently implicated in a particular behavioral disorder that provides a model for human schizophrenia. She uses a new, highly sensitive tract-tracing technique to map this area in rodents that have been genetically engineered to express an altered form of a specific gene. These animals are interesting because they are also deficient in a specific learning task, and this behavioral deficit is quite similar to a behavioral deficit observed in schizophrenic patients. To examine tissue blocks from her experiments for the presence of tracer substances, Dr. Smith uses a microscope connected to a computer workstation, which allows her to record the data onto maps of the brain region and to store all of the data in a digital format. This recording method permits rapid computer visualization of the data in three dimensions.

In her examination, Dr. Smith finds a tiny labeled cell group (area X) embedded in the larger nucleus whose existence has not, to her knowledge, been reported before. While she has the map from her experiment on the video screen, Dr. Smith calls up the three-dimensional anatomical database for this brain region and splits the screen to allow sufficient comparisons of her new map with other maps of the nucleus that have been deposited in the database. She looks at maps from normal animals and maps from genetically engineered animals to see if area X exhibits the same general structure in both groups. One of the maps seems to show a group of cells quite similar to area X. Dr. Smith asks the computer to enlarge that map and show its precise location, compared to her map. (The computer can do this because neuroscientists of the future routinely include with their data maps certain landmark designations that are used to align and bring into conformity maps from different investigators.)

Dr. Smith finds that the two groups of cells are in precisely the same location and that the structures of the cells match. She then types a message, which is automatically forwarded to the scientist who contributed the map, requesting more information about his work. Later that afternoon, Dr. Smith receives a message from Robert Green, who says he had noticed this cell group in certain kinds of labeling experiments but that it was not his primary interest. Nevertheless, he has attached all the data he has regarding this experiment to his message, with an offer to help in any way he can. Dr. Smith electronically thanks Dr. Green and asks him if he is aware of any chemical characterization of these cells. As the reply is negative, Dr. Smith enters the neurochemical database for this region and pulls up maps showing the distribution of a variety of neurotransmitters. She finds a map of the distribution of a particular protein (zeta) that clearly includes area X and, again, asks for more information. A documentary summary appears at the side of the screen describing the identification of protein zeta by antibody techniques. The summary also states that protein zeta has a specific distribution in the brain and that researchers suspect that it affects potassium channels in the cells' membranes, making the channels less likely to open during synaptic transmission. Dr. Smith transfers the references for these observations into her personal reference files and asks if protein zeta has been sequenced. The reply is that it has been partially sequenced by a Dr. Ungaro in Italy and that the partial sequence is available in a special part of the Protein Identification Resource (PIR) reserved for preliminary data. (Dr. Ungaro, like Dr. Green, is pursuing another interest and has deposited the partial sequence for use by other investigators.)

Dr. Smith enters the PIR and calls up the partial sequence for protein zeta on one side of the screen. On the other side, she retrieves information about the gene that has been altered in her experimental animals. The computer displays the base pair sequence for the gene, followed by the RNA sequence for which the gene codes. From the RNA sequence, the computer displays the expected protein sequence. Dr. Smith instructs the computer to run a comparison of the expected protein sequence with the partial sequence of Dr. Ungaro and discovers a strong match. She immediately types a message to Dr. Ungaro regarding this match and says that she would like to follow up on this information. Dr. Ungaro replies that he is happy that the information was useful and that he will amend the PIR entry to reflect the probable match and her plan to pursue further study.

A few weeks pass, during which Dr. Smith completes another group of experiments. Her studies show that cells in area X are responsible for the learning deficits in her genetically engineered animals and that protein zeta is an abnormal form that results from the genetic alteration. The protein disrupts the potassium channels by interfering with cyclic AMP, but a new drug that increases the effectiveness of cyclic AMP blocks this effect in Dr. Smith's animals. Moreover, this drug completely alleviates the learning deficits in these animals. Dr. Smith submits these data to an electronic journal, transferring her manuscript text, photomicrographs, sequence comparisons, and other data directly from her computer to the journal. The journal electronically transmits the manuscript to reviewers. Eventually, the manuscript is published in electronic and conventional formats, and the accompanying data are deposited into the appropriate databases. Work in other laboratories then begins to document the biochemical mechanisms that have been discovered and the new drug's effectiveness in human schizophrenics.

As new experiments proceed, Dr. Ungaro's protein is finally sequenced, and this information, along with Dr. Smith's data, is moved by PIR's editors from the preliminary data files of the PIR into its main files of verified data. Dr. Green's contribution is acknowledged in the manuscript and in the anatomical brain database. Such documentation is of great use to investigators who have become interested in protein zeta and its role in schizophrenia. A contribution index database keeps track of the results of data deposits such as those of Drs. Green and Ungaro, and such records are often submitted, along with authored publications, to university tenure and promotion committees.

Parts of this scenario could be implemented today; others await further technological, and perhaps sociological, advances. But the useful, coordinated complex of resources suggested in the story will not evolve on its own; it must be planned and put into place. It is the consensus of this committee that now is the time to begin that effort.

Critical Breakthroughs, Important Opportunities

Computers and computer graphics help scientists obtain new images

Neuroscience is an inherently visual science, and in this way it differs from other scientific fields, based on mathematical calculations, that already have benefited from advances in computer science. The widespread use of computers in neuroscience had to wait for major technological breakthroughs in computer graphics, which depended in large measure on increases in the power of individual computers and the associated steep decrease in the cost of that power. In 1945, it cost approximately $1,000 to perform 1 million computer operations. In 1970, the same number of operations cost less than 6 cents; in 1980, they cost 0.1 cent. By 1997, this cost is expected to decrease by a factor of 100. In terms of time, in 1945, 1 million operations took a month; they took 0.1 second in 1980 and, in 1990, in the case of some of the most powerful workstations, roughly 2.5 milliseconds (U.S. Congress, Office of Technology Assessment, 1990). Such trends are continuing in the present decade.

More than power, the memory capabilities of a computer determine its cost. Again, consistent increases in memory, accompanied by decreases in cost, have occurred over the past three decades (Figure 4-1). In 1965, a computer with 64 kilobytes (KB) of memory cost about $200,000 (Bell, 1988) and was used, for example, in expensive satellites and space probes, such as Voyager II. Today, computers of that size cost about $100 and are used to drive popular computer games (e.g., the small, hand-held version of Nintendo®, Gameboy®). Why is a computer capable of running Voyager II necessary for a computer game toy with a tiny video screen? The answer is that the graphics of the toy and the ability to interact with those graphics require far more computer power than is required by calculations (Table 4-1). Today's computer graphics—from the dazzling special effects of movies to the variety of the evening news promotions— could not have been accomplished without the recent improvements in computer hardware and software.

Computer graphics is a subspecialty of computer science pioneered by Ivan Sutherland and others in the early 1960s (Goldberg, 1988). The work of these early investigators and the people they trained led to the development of the first primitive graphics workstation less than 20 years ago. The Association for Computing Machinery, one of two major associations of computer science, has a special-interest graphics group that holds a convention every year. In addition to scientific presentations and workshops, this convention includes seminars on various kinds of graphics applications, a computer graphics art show, and exhibits from numerous computer hardware and software companies. The almost 40,000 who now attend this convention, ranging from Hollywood artists to automotive engineers to defense contractors, are an indication of how pervasive, and accessible, computer graphics have become in industry and government (ACM SIGGRAPH, 1989).

The use of computer graphics in biomedical research is also becoming pervasive (albeit not as quickly as in such fields as earth mapping, physics, and space science) and is evolving into the concept of scientific visualization, sometimes called visualization computing (National Academy of Sciences, 1989). In 1987 the National

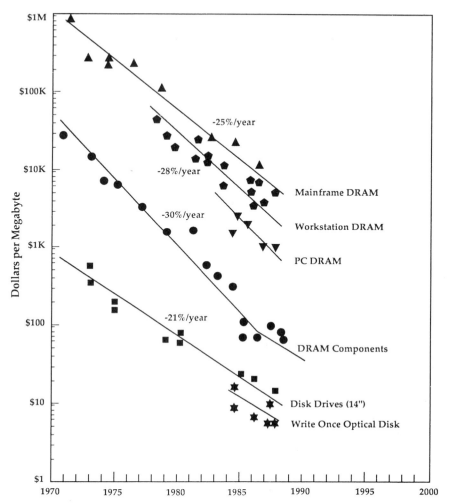

FIGURE 4-1 The cost (in dollars) of computer memory (in megabytes), which has decreased steadily since 1970. DRAM = dynamic random access memory. Chart provided by Mark Duncan of ASKMAR, derived from a graph by Frank Ura of Hewlett-Packard.

Science Foundation convened a panel to consider scientific visualization in many fields, including biomedical science (McCormick et al., 1987). This panel observed that the human eye recognizes geometric and spatial relationships faster than it recognizes other relationships and that the visual display of data would be more efficient for human pattern recognition than displays of numbers and text. Thus, visual-

TABLE 4-1 Text Versus Image Data: Byte Requirements

Application	Example	Approximate No. of Bytes Required
Word processing	One computer screen of text, 25 rows × 80 characters/row	2,000 (2 KB)
Image processing		
Low-end[a]	Magnetic resonance and computed tomography images	262,144 (256 KB; 100 times more information than a screenful of text)
High-end[b]	Computer-aided design (CAD; architecture and engineering applications)	1,310,720 (1.25 MB)
Volumetric Imaging[c]	Realistic three-dimensional images with shadows, highlights, reflections, and transparencies	4,294,967,296 (4 gigabytes; 16,000 times more information than a magnetic resonance or computed tomography image)

Abbreviations:

Bit = binary digit, of which there are only two possible: 0 and 1;
Byte = the number of bits (usually 8) that represent one character;
Kilobyte (KB) = 1,024 bytes;
Megabyte (MB) = approximately 1 million bytes;
Gigabyte = approximately 1 billion bytes;
Terabyte = approximately one trillion bytes.

[a]512 × 512 pixel display (8 bits/pixel).
[b]1280 × 1024 pixel display (8 bits/pixel).
[c]1K × 1K × 1K voxel display (32 bits/voxel).

ization computing draws on computer graphics, image processing, computer-aided design, signal processing, and user interface studies, with the goal of "transforming the symbolic into geometric reality, [and] offering a method to see the unseen" (McCormick et al., 1987).

One of the most successful applications of scientific visualization in biomedical science has been the modeling of molecular structures from data derived from x-ray crystallography. In the past, such structures were inferred from the numerical coordinate data obtained in complex experiments and then drawn by hand or modeled with sticks and balls to represent atoms or other molecular components. These representations depended on the imagination of viewers and their ability to visualize three dimensions from a flat plane and a dynamic image from a static one. Now, computer graphics use mathematical data to generate a moving, dynamic, three-dimensional structure that can change its shape as a consequence of "experimental" conditions entered into the computer or that can be rotated to achieve a different perspective (Plate 4-1). These dynamic computer models are sufficiently similar to the in vivo molecules that they may soon help scientists to predict which drugs might stop viruses, how genes are turned on and off, or how two molecules interact with each other (Howard Hughes Medical Institute, 1990). Not only are these models useful for data analysis but they greatly enhance the communication of research results by making those results much more accessible to scientists and nonscientists alike (U.S. Congress, Science Policy Study, 1986).

Virtually every kind of data used in neuroscience can be collected, stored, analyzed, and visualized on a computer. The raw data from some techniques are already collected directly into computer-readable form. For example, in CT, PET, and MRI scans, the data are collected in the computer as numbers, which the computer uses to form images on its monitors. The images can be displayed in a monochrome scale of gray, or they can be enhanced by assigning colors to certain numerical ranges. In all present-day, computer-based image processing, the numerical data rather than the images are stored, because the images can be recreated from numbers at any time. Increasingly, electrophysiological data and data from EEG and ERP studies are also collected in computer-ready form. Later, the traces of electrical activity can be graphically reconstructed on a computer for analysis (Plate 4-2).

Anatomical data can be computerized in a variety of ways. For example, electron microscopic photographs of brain tissue can be digitized, and regions of these photographs can be analyzed for total surface area or volume using readily available software programs. One group has reconstructed three-dimensional images of the complex innervation patterns of the cells responsible for body equilibrium from a montage of many electron micrographs (Ross et al., 1990). Sections of whole brains have also been digitized and the sections combined in a three-dimensional display so as to allow rotation and slicing of the brain in any plane of section; information regarding neurochemistry or other variables can then be overlaid on specific regions (Plate 4-3; Toga, 1989). An effort to digitize brain sections is under way at the Comparative Mammalian Brain Collection (CMBC), housed at the University of Wisconsin and Michigan State University, to increase the usefulness of this important archival collection (W. Welker, J. Johnson, and S. Greenberg, CMBC, personal communication, 1990). Beyond its uses in basic science, digitization is also important to clinical neuroradiology. When x-rays are transformed into digital files, the images can be reconstructed in distant locations. This relatively easy method of transmitting important medical records has spurred great interest in building a network system to transmit such images among hospitals (Banks et al., 1986; Elliot et al., 1990).

Until recently, researchers were forced to trace individually stained neurons by hand using a special accessory on a light microscope. Now, however, these drawings can be done automatically with a computerized confocal microscope that reconstructs neurons in three dimensions (Figure 4-2). The neuronal images can be studied on their own or used as templates to display differential inputs to specific parts of a neuron. Computer graphics can also be used to display data from pharmacological and neurochemical studies, which normally generate numerical data. The computer can transform numerical measurements, such as dose, response magnitude, and time, into three-dimensional contoured histograms. Such wide-ranging capabilities give investigators unprecedented flexibility in the collection, viewing, analysis, and communication of neuroscience research data.

Increased use of computers in data collection and analysis is apparent from the number of private companies that now market computer hardware and software for neuroscience applications. At the Society for Neuroscience Annual Meeting in 1990, 10 companies exhibited workstations useful for neuroscience research, and 43 companies offered software packages that did almost everything from three-dimensional reconstructions of neurons to quantification and graphic display of fluorescent color changes in ion-sensitive dye experiments. The companies marketing these tools included microscope companies, such as Zeiss and Leitz, as well as traditional computer firms, such as Apple and IBM.

Further evidence of the increasingly important role of scientific visualization in neuroscience comes in the priority given to biomedical computing in universities and government laboratories. For example, Stanford University, Washington University, the University of Pittsburgh, Carnegie Mellon University, and the University of North Carolina, among others, have electrical engineering or computer science departments with sections devoted to the development of technologies, especially graphics and imaging, for biomedical data collection and analysis. Researchers from these departments work in conjunction or in collaboration with counterparts from biomedical departments; some departments also have formal ties to the federally supported supercomputing efforts (Twedt, 1990). At the National Institutes of Health, many individual institutes maintain branches in which com-

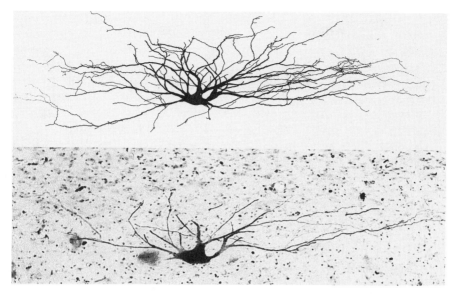

FIGURE 4-2 A spinocervical tract neuron from an adult cat's spinal cord. The lower portion of the figure shows the horseradish peroxidase (HRP)-filled cell that occupies one tissue section. The upper portion is a computer-generated reconstruction from 12 60-micron-thick sections. The cell was identified and stained by M. J. Sedivec, Appalachian State University, and L. M. Mendell, State University of New York, Stony Brook; the reconstruction was performed by J. J. Capowski, Eutectic Electronics, Inc. This photo appeared on the cover of the *Journal of Neuroscience*, March 1986, and was reproduced with permission from Oxford University Press.

puter scientists and software developers work on applications pertinent to the needs of intramural researchers. For example, when a group of researchers at the National Institute of Mental Health (NIMH) developed a new experimental technique and computer software for visualization and image analysis of brain glucose metabolism, the software was freely shared with any investigator interested in using the new technique (Goochee et al., 1980). NIH also maintains a Division of Computer Research and Technology that, in addition to NIH administrative computing oversight, conducts advanced research into such areas as computer modeling of molecular structure, image processing, and scientific workstation development (National Institutes of Health, Division of Computer Research and Technology, 1989). NIH and the National Science Foundation also provide a number of grants to develop useful computer tools for scientific research purposes (National Center for Research Resources, 1990; National Science Foundation, 1991). Finally, the National Library of Medicine (NLM) has developed many easily accessible biomedical databases. In addition, the NLM's Center for Biotechnology Information, in conjunction with its efforts to develop useful scientific databases and database linkages, is concerned with the incorporation of computer graphics as user interface tools (National Library of Medicine, 1986).

Considering the primitive state of computer science, especially computer graphics, only 20 years ago, the contributions of these technologies to the visualization of biological processes are quite remarkable. Future work promises to permit scientists to view data in entirely new ways and to integrate those data to a degree never before possible.

Database technologies help organize our knowledge

A major impact of computer technology has been to enable virtually anyone to collect, store, and access many types of data in digital form and to organize data files into discrete units or collections called databases. Although the term *database* is relatively recent, the concept is as old as symbols carved into clay. The ancient Egyptian records of a grain harvest were databases, as was the census taken by Julius Caesar; the Yellow Pages is a modern example. Computer databases thus reflect the same kind of diversity that other collections of information have shown throughout history. One can classify databases according to what kind of data they contain, how broadly accessible they are, and how formally or informally they are structured (Box 4-1).

Databases can be word, number, image, or sound oriented (Williams, 1990). Word-oriented databases are the most prevalent, and the recent growth in their use has been phenomenal. In 1976 there were 750,000 on-line searches of word-oriented databases (e.g., full-text databases, bibliographic databases, and databases containing information synthesized from numerous sources.) In 1988, however, this number rose to 28.3 billion separate queries (Figure 4-3). Although less common, the use of number-, image-, and sound-oriented databases is also growing. In 1989 there were more than 5,000 databases of all kinds, which were offered by nearly 900 vendors; they contained nearly 5 billion records (compared with 52 million records in 1975). These statistics do not include the hundreds of thousands of private databases in use by individual research scientists for their own purposes.

In terms of accessibility, databases range from entirely public, such as those available on line in libraries, to entirely private, such as

BOX 4-1 RELATIONAL DATABASES VERSUS OBJECT-ORIENTED DATABASES

The database management system most widely in use today is the relational system. In a relational database, information is organized in tables. Many of the tables typically have common fields, allowing the user to associate separate tables and to ask questions about the relationships among different pieces of data. A relational neuroscience database, for example, might include the following two tables: a list of drugs, including their behavioral effects and the types of neurotransmitters through which they exert these effects, and a list of anatomical structures, including the predominant cell type in these structures and the neurotransmitter type associated with these structures. Because these two tables have a field in common (the neurotransmitter field), the database user can ask the computer to briefly link the two tables and to generate a list of drugs and their predominant anatomical sites of action.

One of the major advantages of a relational system is that each piece of data must only be entered once, thus reducing the possibility of error on the initial entry and when updating is required. Should new research indicate that cocaine, for example, exerts its effects by acting on two neurotransmitter systems instead of only one, this new data can be added to the database and will remain linked to all other pieces of information to which it has a relationship. Relational databases are typically used for textual and not for image data.

Database management systems that use object-oriented techniques represent the cutting edge in database technology and are expected to progress rapidly in the coming decade. These systems are designed to support applications with data structures (such as images) that do not fit easily into the table-based structure of the relational system. In an object-oriented system, data need not conform to a standard representation, such as a table, because each piece of data is treated as a separate entity and is stored with its own set of instructions for interacting with other data. This system allows for much greater flexibility in the kinds of data that can be included in a database, and also in the kinds of queries the database can support.

those kept by an individual scientist for his or her own reference. For example, databases printed out on paper or available on floppy or optical disks (e.g., compact-disk, read-only-memory, or CD-ROMs) can be sold or distributed to the public and thus used in any location. *Current Contents*, a popular weekly publication listing the tables of contents of selected scientific journals, is now available in computer-readable form on disks. Other databases might be semiprivate or

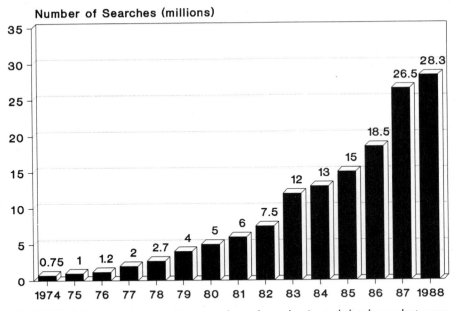

FIGURE 4-3 Growth of on-line searches of word-oriented databases between 1974 and 1988. Adapted from Williams, 1990.

semipublic—shared by a specific group of people—such as several scientists working together on a particular project.

The range of database structures is also broad. Formally structured databases are administered, maintained, updated, and edited in a central location. These databases are generally read-only and include bibliographic reference databases, repositories of historical or archival material, certain types of scientific databases, and directories of various sorts. At the opposite end of the spectrum are informal databases, which are administered, maintained, and updated by users. The user group can be large and membership can be open to everyone, as with the computer bulletin boards that have become so popular. But an informal database can also be structured by a small group of scientists—for example, to keep a "lab notebook" together. Sometimes databases combine both informal and formal components in a unified complex of files. Such a complex might include a bulletin board component, to which users could add data annotations, and a read-only component containing bibliographic reference material. Advances in computer technology make such multicomponent databases feasible by enabling the user to move freely from one component to another. Even entirely separate databases are now collectively accessible by software programs that guide users from one database to another. The flexibility to be gained with the different kinds of databases ensures continuing increases in use patterns.

The growth of biomedical databases mirrors the general trends described earlier. Retrieval of information from the scientific literature is basic to the conduct of biomedical research. Yet over the past 30 years, the number of biomedical investigations, especially in the field of neuroscience, has increased substantially, with many of these efforts branching into related subdisciplines. Computer technology was applied to the management of this expansion by the National Library of Medicine, the lead agency for managing and indexing biomedical and scientific literature. In 1964 the NLM created the Medical Literature Analysis and Retrieval System (MEDLARS), a computerized system that catalogs and indexes the library's holdings. In the early 1970s the NLM introduced MEDLINE, which provides on-line access to NLM's records over telephone lines. Using a carefully formulated and controlled list of key words, known as the Medical Subject Headings (MeSH), users can obtain bibliographic reference lists from MEDLINE for a broad range of scientific topic areas.

Today, in addition to MEDLINE, the NLM offers a number of different kinds of on-line databases of scientific information, including information on toxic substances (TOXLINE and its related databases, the Toxicology Data Bank [TDB] and the Registry of Toxic Effects of Chemical Substances [RTECS]) and medical information related to cancer (the Physician Data Query, or PDQ), among others. Databases such as TDB and PDQ, which are often called factual databases, are more than simply bibliographic records because they contain synthesized information from a variety of sources (National Library of Medicine, 1986). The NLM collaborates with other parts of NIH, with universities, and with other research initiatives to develop a broad range of databases for scientific research and medical practice, to establish directories of these resources, and to design useful interfaces among them. In its long-range plan, articulated in 1986, the NLM defined a number of trends for the future, including databases containing image data, full-text storage and retrieval, and electronic publishing of scientific literature.

Especially prominent among the biomedical databases developed outside of the NLM are the protein sequence and genome databases, which serve at least 23,000 scientists (Table 4-2). These databases provide a mechanism by which extensive, complicated sequence and structural data can be compared to what is already known. Comparisons using such databases are many times more efficient than compari-

TABLE 4-2 Selected Genome and Scientific Databases

Database	Date Established	Kinds of Data	Size
Protein Identification Resource (PIR) National Biomedical Research Foundation Georgetown University Washington, D.C.	Early 1970s	All completely sequenced proteins; amino-terminal sequences and fragmentary sequence data for numerous types of proteins for which sequences are unavailable; bibliographic citations	9,000 Entries
Protein Data Bank (PDB) Brookhaven National Laboratory Upton, New York	1973	Atomic coordinates and partial bond connectivities as derived from crystallographic studies; structure factor and phase data for some structures; associated textual information and bibliographic citations	400 sets of atomic coordinates and 100+ sets of structure factors and phases
Genetic Sequence Data Bank (GenBank) Intelligenetics, Inc. Mountain View, California/ Los Alamos National Laboratory Los Alamos, New Mexico	1979	All reported nucleic acid sequences, catalogued and annotated for sites of biological significance in man	10,000 Records
On-line Mendelian Inheritance in Man (OMIM) Welch Medical Library Johns Hopkins University Baltimore, Maryland	1987	Full-text and bibliographic information on known inherited human traits and disorders; linked to gene map and molecular defects in Mendelian disorders list; linked to GDB	Data on more than 5,000 traits and disorders
Chemical Abstracts Service Source Index (CASSI) American Chemical Society Chemical Abstracts Service (CAS) Columbus, Ohio	Early 1970s	Complete bibliographic descriptions of more than 60,000 serials and nonserials monitored by the CAS (1830–present); guides to depositories of unpublished data; holdings information for numerous U.S. libraries and several libraries abroad	400 Billion bytes
Genome Data Base (GDB) Welch Medical Library Johns Hopkins University Baltimore, Maryland	1990	Mapping database—contains chromosome band locations, genes, anonymous DNA segments, fragile sites, DNA probes, and links to source data (e.g., bibliographic references, personal communications, and conference abstracts); extensions to include genetic linkage and order information from various mapping methods; linked to OMIM	Data on 2,000 genes, 6,000 mapped D-segments, and 20,000 references

SOURCE: Vela, 1990, and Williams, 1990.

sons done by hand and have resulted in new discoveries by database users (see Box 2-1). These databases are also a valuable source of experience and knowledge for those involved in developing analogous resources for neuroscience. For example, each of the protein sequence and genome databases was developed independently, often by an individual scientist, and each has a different history of funding, administration, oversight, software development, and data organization (Smith, 1990; Vela, 1990). Although efforts are now under way to integrate these databases, such integration is not without considerable difficulty and expense.

Ideally, users should be able to access information from a number of protein or genome databases, but currently this is impossible because independent development has resulted in quite separate database structures. For example, some of the early databases (e.g., the Protein Identification Resource [PIR] and the Protein Data Bank [PDB]) were developed from isolated files of information without the use of a database management system for indexing and retrieving entries. This strategy worked only as long as the number of entries was relatively small and the databases stood alone. Present efforts to link the PIR and PDB must first establish a database management system for each and create links between the two database environments. The National Center for Biotechnology Information at the NLM is devising linkage software that will make PIR and the Genetic Sequence Data Bank (GenBank) accessible by similar means and commands. GenBank has also been working to strengthen its links to the European Molecular Biology Library (EMBL) and the Japanese DNA Data Bank. In contrast, the Genome Data Base (GDB) at Johns Hopkins has planned for linkages to other databases from its inception.

The databases also display important differences in software development and the availability of analytical tools. PIR includes some analytical software, whereas PDB makes only the code available for analysis, which often leaves the user confronted with unfamiliar software. Other databases, such as GenBank, spend up to 50 percent of their budgets to develop software for analytical purposes and for database conversion to more modern management systems. Making these conversions is time consuming and costly, but also necessary to extract the most useful information from these resources.

The protein sequence and genome databases reflect a variety of funding mechanisms. GenBank, a collaborative project of Los Alamos National Laboratory and Intelligenetics, Inc., is supported by the broadest range of sources, including the National Science Foundation (NSF); the Departments of Defense, Energy, and Agriculture; and NIH, through the NLM, the National Center for Research Resources, and the National Institute of General Medical Sciences. PDB receives funds from NSF, NLM, and DOE. The Howard Hughes Medical Institute, a private agency, currently funds the GDB and the On-line Mendelian Inheritance in Man (OMIM) database. However, in the near future, GDB and OMIM will be supported by federal funding.

In an effort sponsored in part by the NSF and NLM, the Corporation for National Research Initiatives is developing an experimental National Digital Library System (DLS). The initial target databases are MEDLARS and the GDB and OMIM systems at Johns Hopkins University. DLS will network these databases and employ "knowledge robots" (knowbots®)[1] to initiate and manage complex, multiple-database searches. This system makes it unnecessary for users to know any details of how to search a database, where the database is located, or even how many different databases exist (Cerf and Kahn, 1988).

It is clear that much can be learned from the experiences of the protein and genome databases. But as noted in the previous chapter, neuroscience data differ significantly from protein and gene sequence data and present complex problems in terms of three-dimensional displays and integration across varied data types. Despite the growing use of database technology in individual neuroscience laboratories, relatively few steps have been taken to construct databases for general use by neuroscientists. Understandably, most neuroscience databases either target specific regions of the brain, or are designed as an organizational system (to which data can be added by the user) or as a method for making archival data more accessible. Some of the neuroscience database development efforts receive targeted funding; others do not. These efforts are important because they demonstrate a growing scientific need and address the various kinds of data inherent in neuroscience, especially images. We describe two such efforts below.

A neuroscience information management system called *Brain Browser* has been developed for use on Macintosh computers by a team of neuroscientists with computer expertise (Bloom, 1989). The system is based on HyperCard®, which organizes information in a relational manner, similar to cross-referenced index cards. Contained within the system is information regarding 300 brain regions in the rat, including 900 separate circuits, and references. In addition, the system includes a complete stereotaxic atlas for the rat brain, which can be used as a graphic-based interface to access circuitry data (Figure 4-4). Rather than being a self-contained, read-only system, *Brain Browser* can be expanded by users, who may add "index cards" of their own references and data and customize the database for their own use and that of others (if they share their entries).

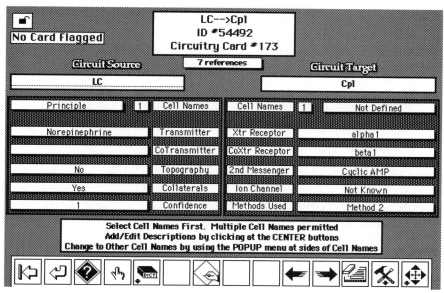

FIGURE 4-4 A typical computer screen from the *Brain Browser* software program. Figure courtesy of Floyd Bloom, Scripps Clinic and Research Foundation. Reprinted with permission of Raven Press.

Another group of neuroscientists and computer scientists from three universities is developing computer tools for high-resolution capture, storage, and organization of neuroscience data (Hillman et al., 1990). Their objective is to construct three-dimensional color atlases, based on real images of brain sections, that are linked to other image, text, and numerical data regarding the anatomy, chemistry, and physiology of specific brain regions. This work is also intended to develop useful software for the extraction of important features and for interfaces that allow transitions from one data type to another. All efforts are focused on one brain region, the thalamic nuclei. Such a focus allows the investigators, who are already expert in thalamic function, to assess more adequately the usefulness and feasibility of the tools being developed.

These two examples may obscure the fact that the development of useful tools to manage neuroscience information is really in its embryonic stages. The majority of neuroscientists use computers for word processing or to organize references and, sometimes, their data images. These are highly individual approaches and vary widely in sophistication. The next section on networks argues that electronic transmission of data sets, including images, most likely will be an integral part of science in the future. Whether neuroscience will be ready for this kind of future depends on the actions taken now to develop the ability to organize data and combine that organization with data collection.

Electronic networks greatly increase communication

The scientific enterprise is composed of men and women who generate ideas, design ways to test those ideas, collect data, and communicate the ideas and data in a variety of ways. The communication of ideas and results is as important to the growth of knowledge as the data themselves. Scientists meet at formal gatherings, discuss experiments with their colleagues, publish papers, and talk to each other by telephone and electronic mail. One of the major goals of computer network development is to create a communication environment that is as free of barriers as possible—an environment that can support the rapid communication of ideas and images at every stage of experimentation and discovery. Some have envisioned this environment as a "National Collaboratory"[2] (Lederberg and Uncapher, 1989). Its cornerstone would be vast networks of electronic links built on a foundation that was begun little more than 20 years ago.

The first multipurpose wide area network (WAN) was developed in 1969 to link computers at 30 research campuses whose work was supported by the Department of Defense. Called ARPANET, the network allowed the sharing of large, expensive computers and facilitated electronic message delivery among widely scattered university and industrial research sites throughout the United States. ARPANET was extremely successful because of a specially developed mechanism for routing messages, called packet switching. Packet switching is unlike the circuit-switching mechanism that connects one telephone to another; no actual circuit is established when a message is sent over a packet-switched network. Rather, the messages are broken up into packets, like envelopes, with address information attached. These packets move from one network node to another, as a letter moves from post office to post office until it reaches its destination. Electronic messages arrive within fractions of seconds, however, not days (Kahn, 1987).

Local area networks (LANs) link computers across short distances (within an office building or among university laboratories, for instance) and are often linked themselves to national and international WANs. Since their introduction in the 1970s, more than 5 million LANs have been installed. In 1973, the Defense Advanced Research Projects Agency (DARPA), which funded the development of ARPANET's packet-switching technology, began a project to develop technology to interconnect different packet-switching networks. A series of computer communication protocols were developed for this purpose, along with "gateways" to interlink different LAN and WAN computer networks. The so-called TCP/IP protocol suite that resulted is used today to interconnect 5,000 networks in 35 countries supporting more than 300,000 computers that range from supercomputers to workstations and even personal computers. The system, which is called the Internet (Quarterman, 1989), is operated on a collaborative, cooperative basis involving government, military, university, and industrial resources and thousands of volunteers who keep the system operating.

In 1988, the National Science Foundation began work on the NSFNET to interconnect a small number of supercomputer centers and to sponsor the creation of intermediate-level, or regional, networks to provide access to the NSFNET and its supercomputing resources. Some 13 supercomputer centers and 400 universities are linked to the NSFNET, along with more than 2,000 other networks whose traffic the NSFNET supports. The NSFNET and its "entourage" are now an integral, vital component of the international Internet.

The full utility of such large-scale networking can be realized only if standards are established to enable effective communication among the computer systems that constitute the network (National Academy of Sciences, 1989). The Internet Activities Board and its subsidiary groups, the Internet Research and Engineering Task Forces, are responsible for guiding research and development of standard protocols for Internet computer communication. The quest for useful, yet practical, standards for the communication of numeric, text, image, and other signals data continues and could play an important role in the creation of an effective national neural circuitry database.

One of the most critical limitations of networks for scientific applications is the capacity, or bandwidth, of the present links. Bandwidth refers to the amount of data that can be transmitted per second. For example, NSFNET began with links capable of transmitting 56 kilobits of information per second. A full-text article from a scientific journal averages 20 kilobytes, or 160 kilobits; an abstract averages 16 kilobits. Thus, NSFNET's initial bandwidth was sufficient to transmit three to four abstracts, but not even one entire journal article, per second. In 1989, NSFNET upgraded its system to links capable of transmitting 1.5 megabits per second—large enough for 10 full-text articles or approximately 100 abstracts. Upgrades now in progress will increase the NSFNET backbone-link bandwidth to 44.7 megabits per second, almost a 30-fold increase in the amount of information transmitted every second. Traffic in the NSFNET backbone has reached nearly 5 billion packets per month, and the rate of increase is still substantial. The introduction of 45 megabit-per-second capability into the NSFNET is an intermediate step in the race toward gigabit-(a billion bits)-per-second service, which will be needed as communication of image data becomes more prevalent.

A single line drawing or simple black-and-white picture represents the same amount of data as an entire journal article of text. An uncompressed transmission rate of 180 megabits per second is required to run a color movie on a conventional TV screen in real time. Computer-generated images on high-resolution screens require much more: 1.44×10^9 bits per second. Consequently, for useful multimedia network transmission, transmission rates will have to reach at least the gigabit-per-second range or higher. (A gigabit equals the information contained in 80,000 double-spaced pages of text.)

The importance of building a nationwide high-bandwidth network is underscored by the attention such a network is receiving from policymakers. An early proposal for a nationwide system of electronic links among supercomputers and libraries was made by Senator Albert Gore in 1979, and the resulting legislation was considered by Congress in 1990 and is being reintroduced this year (Gore, 1990). In 1985, Congress passed Senator Gore's Supercomputer Network Study Act, authorizing the Office of Science and Technology Policy (OSTP) to analyze the need for such a network. Citing the lack of adequate network technology for "scientific collaboration or access to unique scientific resources" and the aggressive efforts of Japan and Europe to upgrade their networks, the OSTP report, issued in 1987, strongly recommended that federal resources be allocated to upgrade existing networks and undertake the research necessary to advance network technology even farther. In 1988, the National Research Council's National Research Network Review Committee issued a report that expanded the specific recommendations made by OSTP but also strongly recommended the implementation of a National Research Network. This recommendation was strongly endorsed in 1989 by the National Academy of Sciences' Panel on Information Technology and the Conduct of Research (National Academy of Sciences, 1989). A further indication of the attention being devoted to this issue was a report entitled *The Federal High Performance Computing Program*, delivered to Congress in 1989 by the President's science advisor, D. Allan Bromley (Office of Science and Technology Policy, 1989). This program plan again recommended a phased development of a National Research and Education Network, now commonly called NREN. Three major objectives specified by all of these initiatives were (1) to upgrade the bandwidth of the backbone networks currently serving science and education to at least gigabit-per-second speed beginning in the mid- to late 1990s; (2) to develop appropriate technology and communication standards that would significantly improve the ability to communicate over electronic networks; and (3) to increase the ubiquity of networking (the NREN program, in particular, proposes to establish connectivity between 1,000 research and education institutions).

Some electronic collaboratory groups are forming now

A critical mass of enthusiasm has been building among legislators, policymakers, and scientists about the possibilities offered by network technology to provide an infrastructure for enhanced scientific collaboration. An interesting project to realize the collaboratory concept is now under way (Schatz, 1991). The project's objectives are to encode, in digital form, all knowledge of the community of biologists who study the worm *Caenorhabditis elegans* and to construct an integrated computer environment to manipulate this knowledge across the Internet. There are about 500 scientists in this multidisciplinary "worm community," representing genetics, anatomy, physiology, biochemistry, and neuroscience, and the community has always had a high degree of openness in communication and data sharing. For example, for more than a decade, the group has maintained a newsletter of news and research findings to which anyone may contribute. On numerous occasions, the newsletter has reported significant research in advance of formal publication, thus functioning as an electronic bulletin board.

Genetic mapping is a major aim of the worm community, as it is of many scientists engaged in the study of invertebrate models (National Research Council, 1985). Alan Coulson and John Sulston have already established a physical map database of *C. elegans* genes, using DNA fragments that they made or that were sent to them by other researchers (Coulson et al., 1986). About 70 percent of the worm's 100 million-base-pair genome has been mapped thus far. This information, updated monthly through Bitnet and Internet, is contained within a digital database that is distributed to several sites; from there, the database can be accessed by modem or direct electronic connection by any worm laboratory.

The current initiative intends to draw on the successful experience of the physical map database and newsletter to build an electronic worm community. Plans include making the entire body of *C. elegans* knowledge available in digital form and constructing strong electronic platforms for informal communication and to support powerful analysis and annotation, as well as retrieval. This project in many ways could be a "test bed" for neuroscience because it involves the conversion of many types of data into digital forms suitable for inclusion in a coordinated, multimedia research resource. For example, so much is known about the neurons that make up the worm's nervous system that each neuron's developmental lineage, wiring diagram, and physical location are understood. The organization of this neural information into a mixed text-numerical-image database would be of tremendous value to future work with data from more complicated organisms.

The openness of the worm community offers another important model for developers of computerized resources for neuroscience because a major portion of the current project involves the inclusion of informal data in the database and the establishment of electronic means of communication. These informal data include everything from recipes for laboratory reagents to intermediate experimental results. How the various kinds of informal data are handled, how continued openness is encouraged and rewarded, and how interfaces are designed for the most efficient use of resources by the community will be applicable in the larger context of neuroscience. Most important, because the worm community cannot answer all the questions posed by the incorporation of these technologies into the field of neuroscience, consideration of the worm community's efforts will help to focus the design of specific pilot projects in the larger neuroscience context.

Conclusion

The role of electronic networks in biomedical science can be expected to expand as network capabilities are upgraded. With these upgrades and the implementation of such projects as the National Digital Library System and the worm community initiative, the formation of national or international collaboratories becomes a more realistic goal for many fields of science. For neuroscience, high-resolution computer imaging and high-bandwidth networking are converging, and major obstacles to the integration of enabling technologies in the research enterprise are quickly diminishing. By beginning now, the integration of these technologies into neuroscience will be ensured. As an added benefit, integrating these technologies into a field as complex as neuroscience will help to generate new ways of conducting scientific exploration that will be applicable to all of biomedical and biological science.

References

ACM SIGGRAPH. 1989. Computer Graphics: SIGGRAPH '89 Conference Proceedings 23(3).

Banks, G., J. K. Vries, and S. McLinden. 1986. Radiologic automated diagnosis. IEEE 195:228-239.

Bell, C. G. 1988. Toward a history of (personal) workstations. Pp. 1-47 in A History of Personal Workstations, A. Goldberg, ed. New York: ACM Press.

Bloom, F. 1989. Databases of brain information. Chapter 13 in Three-Dimensional Neuroimaging, A. Toga, ed. New York: Raven Press.

Capowski, J. J., M. J. Sedivec, and L. M. Mendell. 1986. An illustration of spinocervical tract cells and their computer reconstruction (cover). Journal of Neuroscience 6(3).

Cerf, V., and R. Kahn. 1988. The Digital Library System: The World of Knowbots, vol. 1. Reston, Va.: Corporation for National Research Initiatives.

Coulson, A., J. Sulston, S. Brenner, and J. Karn. 1986. Towards a physical map of the genome of the nematode Caenorhabditis elegans. Proceedings of the National Academy of Sciences USA 83:7821-7825.

Elliot, L. P., S. K. Mun, S. C. Horii, and H. Benson. 1990. Digital Imaging Network System (DINS) Evaluation Report. Washington, D.C.: Department of Radiology, Georgetown University Medical Center.

Goldberg, A., ed. 1988. A History of Personal Workstations. New York: ACM Press.

Goochee, C., W. Rasband and L. Sokoloff. 1980. Computerized densitometry and color coding of [14C] deoxyglucose autoradiographs. Annals of Neurology 7(4):359-370.

Gore, A. 1990. Networking the future. Washington Post, July 15.

Hillman, D. E., R. R. Llinas, M. Canaday, and G. Mahoney. 1990. Concepts and methods of image acquisition, frame processing, and image data presentation. Pp. 3-38 in Three-Dimensional Neuroimaging, A. Toga, ed. New York: Raven Press.

Howard Hughes Medical Institute. 1990. Finding the Critical Shapes. Bethesda, Md.: Howard Hughes Medical Institute Office of Communications.

Kahn, R. E. 1987. Networks for advanced computing. Scientific American 257:136-143.

Lederberg, J., and K. Uncapher, co-chairs. 1989. Towards a National Collaboratory: Report of an Invitational Workshop. Rockefeller University, New York City, March 17-18.

McCormick, B. H., T. A. DeFanti, and M. D. Brown, eds. 1987 Visualization in scientific computing. SIGGRAPH Computer Graphics Newsletter 21(6):1-13.

National Academy of Sciences. 1989. Information Technology and the Conduct of Research. Washington, D.C.: National Academy Press.

National Center for Research Resources. 1990. Biomedical Research Technology Resources: A Research Directory. Pub. No. 90-1430. Bethesda, Md.: National Institutes of Health.

National Institutes of Health, Division of Computer Research and Technology. 1989 Annual Report. Bethesda, Md.: National Institutes of Health.

National Library of Medicine. 1986. Obtaining Factual Information from Data Bases: Report of Long Range Planning Panel 3. Bethesda, Md.: National Institutes of Health.

National Research Council. 1985. Models for Biomedical Research: A New Perspective. Washington, D.C.: National Academy Press.

National Research Council. 1988. Toward a National Research Network. Washington, D.C.: National Academy Press.

National Science Foundation. 1991. Guide to Programs. Pub. No. 038-000-00585-5. Washington, D.C.: U.S. Government Printing Office.

Office of Science and Technology Policy, Executive Office of the President. 1987. A Research and Development Strategy for High Performance Computing. Washington, D.C. November 20.

Office of Science and Technology Policy, Executive Office of the President. 1989. The Federal High Performance Computing Program. Washington, D.C. September 8.

Quarterman, J. S. 1989. The Matrix. New York: Digital Press.

Ross, M. D., L. Cutler, G. Meyer, T. Lam, and P. Vaziri. 1990. 3-D components of a biological neural network visualized in computer generated imagery. Acta Otolaryngologia (Stockholm) 109:83-92.

Schatz, B. R. 1991. Building an Electronic Scientific Community. Pp. 739-748 in Proceedings of the 24th Annual Hawaii International Conference on System Sciences, IEEE Computer Society, vol. 3.

Smith, T. F. 1990. The history of the genetic sequence databases. Genomics 6:701-707.

Toga, A., ed. 1989. Three-Dimensional Neuroimaging. New York: Raven Press.

Twedt, S. 1990. Biologists find speed, imaging powers of supercomputers key to research. The Scientist (Aug. 20):10-11.

U.S. Congress, Office of Technology Assessment. 1990. Critical Connections: Communication for the Future. OTA-CIT-407. Washington, D.C.: U.S. Government Printing Office.

United States Congress, Science Policy Study. 1986. The Impact of the Information Age on Science. Hearings, vol. 10. Pub. No. 57-0950. Washington, D.C.: U.S. Government Printing Office.

Vela, C. 1990. Overview of U.S. Genome and Selected Scientific Databases. Background paper prepared for the Committee on a National Neural Circuitry Database, Institute of Medicine.

Williams, M. E. 1990. The state of databases today: 1990. Pp. vii-xiv in Computer-readable Databases: A Directory and Data Sourcebook, K. Y. Marcaccio and J. Adams, eds. Detroit, Mich.: Gale Research, Inc.

Notes

1. Knowbots is a registered trademark of the Corporation for National Research Initiatives.

2. The concept of a national collaboratory does not ignore the essentially international character of science. Responsibility for the infrastructure of each national collaboratory should rest, as it traditionally has, with the governmental agencies of each nation that places a priority on scientific excellence. The international collaboratory would be created simply by establishing links among these national resources.

5

Building Consensus, Identifying Needs

In meeting its charge, the committee consulted more than 150 neuroscientists and computer and information science experts who contributed advice, comments, and suggestions regarding the desirability, feasibility, and possible ways of implementing electronic and digital resources to enhance neuroscience. As outlined in the introduction to this report, the committee obtained these contributions through four mechanisms. The first was the preparation of two background papers. One considered the development, administration, architecture, use patterns, and funding of genome and other scientific databases (Vela, 1990). The other described the results of a one-day meeting of computer scientists from various disciplines who had been involved in the Defense Mapping Agency's (DMA) program to digitize cartographic data (Downs et al., 1990). The meeting was held to assess what could be learned from the DMA's experience that might apply to implementation of a National Neural Circuitry Database.

The second mechanism was the organization of four task forces composed of neuroscientists and computer information specialists. Each of the groups met for two days and were organized around neuroscience topic areas; they included 35 invited participants in addition to specific committee members. (Appendix A contains a description of the themes and a list of participants of each task force.) Third, the committee solicited input from a number of other sources as an additional information mechanism. Letters were sent to the present officers and council members, as well as the past presidents, of the Society for Neuroscience describing the study and inviting opinions and suggestions. Similar descriptions with a request for input were also published in selected scientific journals (for examples, see Appendix B).

Finally, symposia and open hearings were held in Washington, D.C., San Francisco, and Chicago. Invitations to these events were sent to members of the Society for Neuroscience within roughly a 300-mile radius of each meeting location. The program for each meeting included scientific presentations by a leading neuroscientist and by a scientist from the field of genetics or molecular modeling with experience in the use of computer and information technology in their research. Also on the agenda were demonstrations of prototype brain databases and brain imaging technologies. Finally, each meeting included an open hearing component in which selected committee members reviewed some of the issues being considered in the study and subsequently opened the floor to comments and suggestions from those in attendance. (Appendix C contains lists of speakers and demonstrators.)

The input received through these mechanisms reflected a wide variety of experiences and outlooks. Among the neuroscientists involved, some were already committed to the development of computer resources for research purposes, some had no such commitment and were more neutral, and some were frankly skeptical. In addition, they held a variety of posts, ranging from journal editors to postdoctoral fellows and from those employed in large laboratories to those working in single-person operations. Individuals in charge of library resources, scientific database administration and design, and biomedical computer applications were especially valuable participants. Each subdiscipline of computer science—including database design, graphics, software development, networks, and hardware design—was represented. In addition, participants came from academic departments, government laboratories, and private industry.

Some separation of the topics covered in each of these information-gathering activities was apparent. Participants in the open hearings and those who responded to the committee's requests for opinions were concerned largely with three issues: (1) the kind of database and the kinds of data that would be useful to them in their research, (2) the possible institution of standard methods of data collection, and (3) funding of the proposed project. In addition to these matters, task forces devoted substantial time to technical issues and administration, oversight, and implementation strategies. This chapter attempts to capture the richness of the discussions that took place throughout these activities and outlines the data on which the committee's recommendations are based.

Building a Useful Resource Complex

The data that are included must be useful to neuroscientists

The complexity of neuroscience dictates that the scope of the data included in any complex of computerized resources eventually must be quite broad. Although most participants viewed the establishment of such resources as desirable, some felt that traditional archives of neuroscience information (e.g., libraries and journals) were adequate, thus obviating the need to expend scarce funds on computerized information complexes. These dissenting views were countered by evidence, presented by experts from medical libraries and scientific databases, that clearly indicated an integral role for computerized data storage and retrieval, including the linking of scientific databases, in future library services. The majority of those giving input to the committee envisioned the proposed complex of resources as necessarily containing more kinds of information than are now or could in the future be contained in library reference materials and published journals. For example, a journal article, available from the library in full-text format with data graphs and figures, rarely presents all the data that are available—data that could be included in a digital format. A graphically formatted synthesis could greatly facilitate understanding by making the information visual. In addition, archival brain material, such as that contained in the Yakovlev brain collection or the Comparative Mammalian Brain Collection, is not available at all in libraries; it could be made much more accessible through electronic networks and digital storage methods. Finally, the vision of a complex of resources for neuroscience includes the incorporation of informal data, such as preliminary results and interpretations, which would provide a far richer base of information for research than is currently available. (Although later sections of this chapter expand upon these nontraditional kinds of information, they are mentioned here as components of the data that may be included in the proposed resource complex.)

Given the vision of resources that go well beyond what may reasonably be obtained from libraries, nearly every participant had an idea of what kinds of research data would be most useful. Although these suggestions reflected a broad range of possibilities, most participants saw two major data categories as critical. The organizing structure for information about the brain is neuroanatomy, which provides a construct for the functional expression of brain activity. Therefore, it will be necessary to conjoin anatomy and function, and this combination should guide decisions regarding the inclusion of highly specific kinds of data.

Primary among the anatomical data categories is information about the pathways that interconnect brain regions. Representing such pathways in three dimensions and in relation to standard brain atlas maps is highly desirable and can serve a number of purposes. Viewing a particular pathway allows an immediate appreciation of its complexity and may reveal the connections among specific areas of interest. Depiction of those parts of the pathway that are well documented as well as those parts that are tentative or unknown would stimulate additional research to complete the mapping of the pathway. The pathway map could also serve as an interface or entry point to archives of relevant bibliographic references.

Most important, a pathway map could function as the skeleton on which to hang information from multiple levels of the brain's hierarchy. For example, at the cellular level of the hierarchy, the structural features or morphology of different cell types are important. Because each brain region contains sets of neurons with different structures, it is often important to know which structural type actually contributes to a pathway to a distant brain region and which structural type contributes only local connections. The neurochemistry of the neurons in the pathway is also of interest at both the cellular and the systems levels. Therefore, a number of participants requested that the proposed resource complex support the ability to associate patterns of neurotransmitter distribution with structural pathways. One scientist suggested that both visual and tabular maps of the chemical systems of the brain would be of great help in his work. Such maps would include the neurotransmitters, as well as the distribution of specific receptor types and of drug binding sites in the brain.

There was consensus that any anatomical map must be related to function, but the functions requested reflected the hierarchical level at which individual scientists were working. Those studying cognitive processing and human brain functions viewed the association of brain regions with specific aspects of behavior as necessary to the usefulness of the map. Clinical neuroscientists were interested in the association of behaviors (e.g., tremor, memory dysfunctions, motor deficits) with particular brain regions. Basic researchers, studying the electrophysiological responses of individual neurons or single-ion channel responses, wanted the map to contain information about these phenomena. Enthusiasm for including many kinds of synaptic-level information was especially high among computational neuroscientists, which reflects their interest in analyzing the functional consequences of ion channel diversity, in terms of the nonuniform spatial distribution of channels and the varied response properties of individual channels. Finally, some investigators interested in the development of the nervous system saw particular benefits in including brain maps of different species at different developmental points as a way of comparing species.

Other kinds of data that were cited as central to neuroscience research were protein and gene sequence and gene mapping data relevant to the brain. Many developmental neuroscientists, through the use of simple organisms such as worms and fruit flies, are now mapping the genes that control neural development. As the genes that code for receptors and other molecules are identified, these data become useful for researchers at other levels of the neural hierarchy. Recent breakthroughs in identifying the genes responsible for such diseases as muscular dystrophy and neurofibromatosis herald a new era in defining the underlying causes of neural dysfunction. Against this backdrop, most task force participants felt a pressing need to include genetic information in any future computerized resource. Their suggestions ranged from the establishment of linkages to existing genome databases to establishment of a brain-specific gene database.

Although the examples given above are not exhaustive of all the suggestions made to the committee, they illustrate the necessity, in the long term, of including specific kinds of data at each level of the neural hierarchy and the appropriateness of starting with the structural anatomy of the brain.

Computerized resources must include a variety of capabilities

Acceptance and full use of computerized resources require certain features or capabilities, apart from the actual data. For example, in molecular modeling, the data are the coordinates obtained from crystallographic analysis. A useful computerized resource must include the capability to transform those coordinates into three-dimensional images and, further, to move these figures to depict the binding of drugs to the molecule's active site. This capability is afforded by the design of the software and the interfaces the user manipulates to achieve the desired outcome. For neuroscience, the capabilities needed will again reflect the diversity of experimental questions that can be asked. Although it is impossible to separate completely the scope of the data to be included from the capabilities of the systems that might be designed, many participants, especially those with expertise in database development, stressed the value of defining desired capabilities early in the planning stages.

Many of the participants providing input to the committee were experienced in the development of prototype systems for research or education, and this group suggested that certain capabilities were essential. For example, the ability to browse through various kinds of data is critical to offering users multiple entry points to access information specific to their needs. Simultaneous display of textual and graphic data or textual and numerical data was also suggested as a necessary feature. These capabilities alone, however, may not be sufficient to ensure use of the proposed resources to their full potential. Therefore, the committee and participants discussed more specific features, designed around the needs of neuroscientists from different subspecialties.

From the neuroscientists' point of view, an important systems capability was the display of data with varied levels of realism. For example, a neuron can be depicted as (1) a photomicrograph (taken through the microscope), (2) a two-dimensional (flat) line drawing, or (3) a fully reconstructed three-dimensional object. If a researcher were interested simply in identifying the cell type, the abstract, flat drawing might suffice. But if he or she were interested in assessing the method used in a particular experiment and in whether the neuron exhibited any changes indicative of injury, the actual photomicrograph might be necessary. In the ideal case, users could choose the level of abstraction appropriate to their experimental needs.

Another capability requested by neuroscientists was the ability to extract arbitrarily defined subsets of data. Using the pathway map as an example, an investigator might want to know the locations of all cells in the pathway that contained a specific neurotransmitter— acetylcholine, for example. Another might want to see all neurons in the pathway that had axons that branched. Yet another might want to know where in the pathway receptors for a specific drug were located. One participant commented on the sometimes puzzling mismatch between the locations of receptors for a certain neurochemical and the locations of cells that contained that neurotransmitter. In his view, the ability to extract receptor and transmitter information and to correlate the two maps would be quite useful. In another neuroscientist's view, the results of computational modeling were a data set well worth extracting. By displaying simultaneously the activity of multiple circuits, it is possible to visualize parallel processing in action.

Another helpful feature for clinical neuroscientists and those involved in human imaging is the ability to compare different brain images by precise overlaying or co-registration of the images. Each brain differs from every other in its exact shape and internal organization. In addition, technical factors, such as how a PET scanner is aligned or the placement of the subject's head, can affect the orientation of the images that are obtained. Schemes for minimizing or correcting for these differences, to facilitate the comparison of different types of images (PET, MR, or CT), have been developed and are being evaluated in most major imaging centers. The task force concerned with human imaging discussed these strategies at length, which include the use of certain landmarks visible in every brain and the use of atlases that describe coordinates for most major brain regions. More complex approaches use experimentally defined algorithms to "warp" one brain image to another. Once these mechanisms are validated, their inclusion, as tools, in a complex of computerized resources would allow investigators to pool images, obtain more data, and thereby gain the maximum benefit from each experiment. Because human subjects are rare and imaging experiments costly, this kind of capability is particularly desirable. Efforts are already under way to share human images among distant centers. Known as BrainMap, the activity is being coordinated by a team of investigators at the Johns Hopkins University Medical School (*Science*, 1990).

Whatever capabilities the proposed complex of resources might include, the consensus of participants in the committee's consultation process was that these features must be defined by the needs of the users. Many participants emphasized the need for a hands-on effort to generate a comprehensive list of desired capabilities.

Different types of databases are required

There was an overwhelming consensus among all participants that a National Neural Circuitry Database as a single entity was unworkable. Participants advocated instead a complex of different kinds of databases, combined with electronic communication facilities and other on-line research tools, that would be interlinked to provide a resource for neuroscience research, education, and clinical applications. In addition, a number of investigators, citing the international character of science, called for the establishment of links to and relationships with computerized resources outside the United States. Throughout the task force meetings and open hearings, there was substantial discussion of the kinds of databases that would be of use to neuroscience. It was the task forces, however, that gave the matter its most in-depth consideration. Consequently, the definitions that follow derive largely from task force recommendations. This emphasis on their work is probably a result of the special efforts made to include in these groups individuals with expertise in database administration and development, as well as those with interest in the concept of electronic collaboratories.

One general theme that emerged was that a complex of electronic and digital resources should include databases with varied levels of accessibility. Some of the databases should be public resources and accessible by anyone; others should be private and used only by individual investigators or small groups. Still others should be semi-private or semipublic, for use by a possibly large, but finite, group of investigators. Within those general categories, the task forces identified several different kinds of databases that are expected to be useful for neuroscience.

- **Reference databases** would contain references to published journal reports and review papers and would be accessible to as wide a group of users as possible. These databases might be built on the kind of information contained in more traditional databases, such as MED-LINE, but they would be organized around graphic representations of brain structures. The images would represent current consensus views of various brain systems and might also show those areas that required additional research. The committee learned from individuals working with the genome databases that attempts are now being made in that community to incorporate graphic representations into those databases. The essentially visual character of neuroscience data underscores the critical importance of images to the presentation of information about the brain.
- **Data banks** would contain source or primary data, with references, that could be deposited by investigators coincident with publication of their research in standard scientific journals. Data banks would allow users to view the complete data set from experiments and might contribute to insights that would not be possible with standard journal formats. These kinds of databases are already in use in the chemical sciences and in the protein and gene sequencing and mapping communities (Vela, 1990).
- **Informal resources** include bulletin boards and electronic mail for exchange of research methods, ideas, and sometimes raw data; these resources might also be used to share software packages. Informal resources are highly flexible and are often designed in response to special user needs. As discussed in the previous chapter, they are an important part of efforts in the worm community to facilitate open communication and exchange (Schatz, 1991).
- **National and international registries or directories** were recommended by each task force and by many other participants to provide listings of different kinds of information. For example, it would be helpful to have a registry of all neuroscientists who are now developing or who have developed computerized data collection strategies, or who have devised databases for storage and retrieval of data, references, or other research information. Among the respondents to the committee's request for opinions and the open hearing participants, approximately 30 individuals were working on databases or

imaging protocols for basic and clinical neuroscience applications—
and the committee had been unaware of their efforts. Another use
for such a registry would be to list data that are available for sharing.

• **Research collaboration databases** are semiprivate or semipublic
databases set up by defined groups of investigators for work on specific projects. Such databases would contain raw data files, methods descriptions, and other information useful to the conduct of the project.
A preliminary survey of long-distance collaborative activities in neuroscience carried out by study staff reinforced the recommendations
of the task forces regarding this kind of database.[1] The survey revealed that approximately 25 percent of all papers published in one
year in *Brain Research* and the *Journal of Neuroscience* were reports of
collaborative work done by two or more geographically distant U.S.
laboratories. Further, study staff asked 10 randomly chosen investigators from these groups if electronic communication facilities, including image transmission, would have helped their work. All
responded in the affirmative.

• **Specialty databases** can also be set up by defined groups. For
example, Task Force 3 (see Appendix A) suggested that such a database would be of great use in brain studies with PET or MR imaging.
If the database were composed of multiple components, including
references, tools for matching or warping one brain image to another,
and a registry of available data, this specialty complex could aid the
transfer of information regarding human brain structure/function
relationships to a wide group of experts.

In summary, this section has outlined some of the key components
of a useful complex of electronic and digital resources, including a
number of different kinds of databases containing information from
all levels of the neural hierarchy. The capabilities afforded by the
complex to browse through the data, compare images, and extract
specific subsets of information would enhance the conduct of neuroscience research and provide assistance extending far beyond what is
now available. But the actual implementation of this complex is a
substantial undertaking, and an understanding of its challenges is
essential for success.

The Challenges Ahead

Technological needs require planning and attention to the most likely advances

Although the current state of computer and information technology has reached a point that makes the proposed complex of com-

puterized resources possible, a number of technical requirements must still be addressed. Such topics received a great deal of attention during the task force deliberations. In the three major areas of databases, networks, and imaging technologies, imaging is the most advanced, from a technological standpoint, and therefore is likely to present the fewest barriers to direct application to neuroscience. Database and network technologies, although sufficiently mature to be applied to neuroscience in a productive manner, will require more modification. To transmit complex images, for example, networks must be upgraded according to the plans formulated for the National Research and Education Network. The task forces were unanimous in their support for careful planning to implement high-bandwidth network links, with special attention to the concomitant upgrades of the local area networks that link researchers inside universities with the national networks. The task forces also emphasized that the use of optical disks or other mass storage media to transmit data physically should be encouraged to obviate complete dependence on network links.

Database management technology presents the most difficult technical challenge in the initial implementation of the proposed resource complex. Currently, the most popular and most useful database design is the relational database; yet these databases cannot meet all of the eventual needs of the neuroscience community because they do not handle image data well and cannot display image and text data simultaneously. Object-oriented database management systems can handle image data, but they may not be widely available during the 1990s. Database developers from the task forces therefore recommended starting with relational models and planning for the eventual conversion to object-oriented systems.

Certain approaches may aid this planning. For example, the Entity Relationship Model is a database design tool that is used to plan the relationships to be set up in a database. In this model, definitions of individual items and their relationships are established before the database is constructed. These definitions are useful to plan both relational and object-oriented management systems. An additional advantage to this approach is that, once completed, it provides a record of the defined relationships, which facilitates later modifications. The model currently is being used at the National Center for Biotechnology Information at the National Library of Medicine in its effort to link Genbank and the Protein Information Resource databases.

Another critical aspect of database design is user interfaces. This area is quickly emerging as a unique subspecialty of computer science, combining human factors research with interface software design and query language development. Interfaces must be easy to use, yet powerful enough to enable the user to extract needed information. Balancing these two qualities is rarely easy, and many task force participants argued for special attention to this issue. They also recommended early involvement of user interface specialists and examination of the experiences of genome database developers in the design of useful interfaces.

Underlying both database and user interface design questions is the challenge of developing software that allows data to be accessible and usable. Indeed, hardware problems are minimal compared with the problems associated with developing software. For example, neuroscientists currently use a variety of computers that run on different operating systems and employ a wide range of software tools; as a result, communication among these systems is severely limited. The task forces made a number of recommendations regarding this problem. One was to develop platform-free software for the databases that would be independent of the operating system being used in the local computing environments and that could circumvent compatibility barriers. However, a better approach might be to design translation programs that could bridge the differences between software programs. In the experience of many participants, software development represents a major portion of the costs associated with database development. Therefore, active encouragement of so-called "shareware" development may produce savings. Shareware is software developed by individuals that subsequently is shared free of charge with others. Examples include software developed in government laboratories, such as that developed for image analysis of results from deoxyglucose experiments (see Chapter 4). The disadvantage of shareware is that often it is not as finely tuned or as carefully maintained as commercially developed software and requires those using it to make modifications for their own needs.

The general theme in the task force software discussions was the advantage of being open to a variety of strategies. Also noted, however, was the need to develop software tools that were directly applicable to research issues. For example, the human imaging group (Task Force 3) identified the need for improvements in the software for registering images with one another. In Task Force 4, participants were acquainted with recent advances by industry and academic research centers in designing software for fast searches of data within a database, including scientific databases. A consensus emerged through these discussions that computer scientists must work in close collaboration with neuroscientists to address the complex problems of software development.

Another area of technological challenge is the mechanism of data storage. Numerous storage options are available, but the choice depends on neuroscientists' needs for specific kinds of data transmission. For example, transmission over networks is compatible with central storage of data in mainframe computers. Because networks currently are inadequate for image transmission, however, transportable media such as optical disks or CD-ROMs are an attractive alternative. Another advantage of transportable storage media is that they may increase accessibility to information, allowing a wider user group, including international users. One computer expert cautioned, however, that the physical organization of the data through these storage mechanisms should not be confused with the logical organization of the data themselves—such confusion would limit access to the data.

The final technical topic covered by the task forces was the development of technical standards for data exchange. The technical issues inherent in standards development are closely related to certain research issues and were of great concern to those who attended the committee's open hearings or contributed written commentary. The issue of standards is explored in the following section.

Standard formats are necessary, but they must evolve

The task forces outlined four categories of technical standards that need to be developed and examined. First, for data representation, standard data exchange formats are required for textual and numerical data and for the generation of images and graphics. Second, for algorithm representation, mechanisms for conveying new algorithms should be considered for a variety of possible applications. Third, standard user-interface packages should be considered as a way to reduce the barriers to the actual use of a given computerized resource. Finally, standard communication protocols should be expanded to provide the dynamic range of data accessibility required for research-oriented databases. Each of these categories reflects the fact that coordinated computer resources require a high level of standardization to function smoothly. Data represented in a multitude of ways, with differing algorithms and with different mechanisms for data access, are often difficult to extract. Communication is further limited by different computing environments and the ability of these environments to accommodate data in forms suitable for transmission.

How database developers approach these technical requirements can have major consequences for the usefulness of the resource. Many neuroscientists who commented on this issue expressed fears that standards might be imposed on them to which they would have difficulty adapting. But the task forces emphasized that standards should evolve from experience and should be based on the needs of users. Their philosophy was that if a standard method or format worked well, usually people were willing to expend a little extra effort to take advantage of the resource for which the standard was designed. In addition, some suggested that establishing liaisons and joint efforts between the neuroscience community and standards development groups (e.g., the standards working groups of the Internet Activities Board) would help to increase awareness in broader user communities of the special requirements of neuroscience data.

The evolution of standards must also begin with an awareness of the specific scientific needs of the user community. One area of concern in neuroscience is that of nomenclature. Disagreements over the names of brain nuclei and subnuclei have been common since the beginning of neuroanatomy. Synonymous terms are widespread but avoidable barriers to communication. A number of participants asked for efforts to establish clear definitions of terms. Others suggested that the NLM expand the Medical Subject Headings (MeSH) in neuroscience subject areas. It might also be worthwhile to follow the lead of the genome databases, which hold regular meetings of user representatives and database managers to discuss nomenclature, as well as other issues.

The committee heard from several neuroscience groups that are already attempting to develop standards. One of these was the imaging community, whose members are seeking effective methods for comparing images. A strategy that is being explored is the general use of an atlas of the human brain as a standard reference frame for expressing neuroanatomical coordinates and regional boundaries. Establishing such a standard might also help to define the range of variability in human brain structure, something that currently is not known. Clinical and basic neuroscientists also suggested standard annotation of experimental data. In human imaging studies aimed at defining structure/function relationships, certain baseline information is now recorded in highly individual ways, which limits its usefulness. At a minimum, such information might include age, handedness, sex, educational level, or any characteristic feature of the subject or experimental group. Basic scientists interested in comparing images (e.g., maps of receptor binding or immunocytochemical localization) asked that images be tied to precise annotative information regarding experimental conditions, calibrations, chemical methods, animal weights, and other appropriate data.

In summary, any discussion of standards touches on technical, scientific, and sociological issues (see National Academy of Sciences, 1989). Although standards development is necessary and cannot be ignored, the clear majority of participants in the committee's consultative process were in favor of allowing most standards to evolve, based on hands-on experience and careful consideration of users' needs. What is critical to keep in mind is that the design of usable standards, which do not involve large investments of individual user's time, will determine, in part, whether an electronic or digital resource will be widely used.

Technology drives sociological change

The sociology of science can be defined as the ways in which scientists work and how they interact. Different scientific fields and subspecialties may display varying sociological attributes. Yet as most of us have witnessed in our everyday lives, the incursion of technology can produce very profound changes in sociological patterns. In each of the committee's consultative activities, from task force meetings to open hearings, the question was asked: How will the incorporation of electronic and digital resources in neuroscience change neuroscience and neuroscientists? The challenge for the future is to understand the technology's possible effects and to begin to develop the policies and approaches necessary to cope with these effects.

One of the advantages of electronic communication and the establishment of informal databases will be the ability to share data with one's colleagues or with the entire community. Data sharing can greatly increase the amount of information gleaned from each experiment and thereby quicken the progress of investigation. In addition to publication of the results of an experiment or study, data sharing could comprise very preliminary data or complete data sets. Yet despite the benefits that can be expected, there are also perceived risks for the investigator wishing to share data (Fienberg et al., 1985; National Academy of Sciences, 1989). One risk is the investment of time in an activity that results in no tangible benefit to the investigator. Methods for assigning credit to scientists who contribute data to databases are rudimentary at present. Because journal publications and other formal mechanisms for assigning credit for specific scientific concepts and results carry substantial weight as benchmarks of an individual's success in science, the matter of proper credit is important. Another risk involves the rights of human research subjects. The strict guidelines that protect the privacy and identity of human research subjects were developed before electronic networks and digital databases were in common use. The sharing of data (e.g., PET and MRI data) obtained from studies of human subjects will require additional

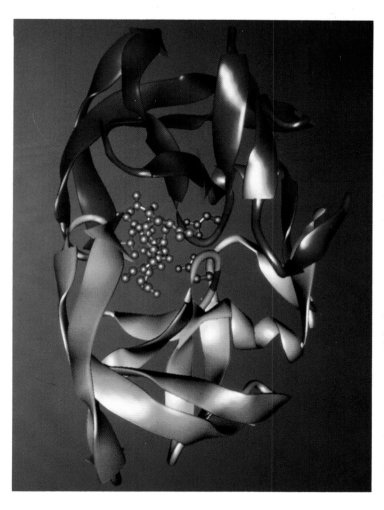

PLATE 4-1 A computer model of an enzyme molecule, the human immunodeficiency virus (HIV-1) protease. The structure was solved by members of the Crystallography Laboratory, National Cancer Institute, Frederick Cancer Research Facility, using synthetic protein supplied by the California Institute of Technology. Molecular graphics by the University of California, San Francisco (UCSF) Computer Graphics Laboratory using UCSF Midas-Plus. Copyright, Regents, University of California. Reprinted with permission.

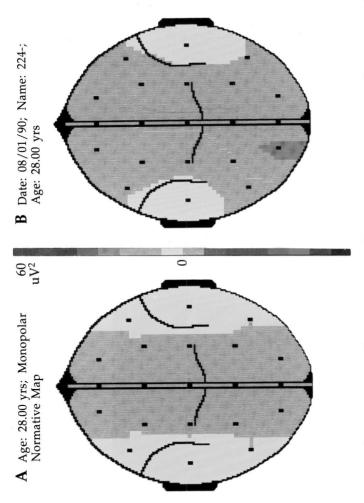

A Age: 28.00 yrs; Monopolar
Normative Map

60
uV²

0

B Date: 08/01/90; Name: 224-;
Age: 28.00 yrs

PLATE 4-2 Computer-assisted reconstruction of EEG activity. Computer software is used to transform an analog EEG signal into quantitative form, in this case, to examine the amplitude of activity of a specific frequency band (the Delta band). The EEG distribution is displayed over the entire scalp (nose is up). The delta power distribution of a normal person is seen in **A** while **B** shows the result obtained in a patient with an aneurysm of the left posterior communicating artery. Figure provided by M. E. Sumas and P. G. Newlon, Department of Neurosurgery, Eastern Virginia Medical School, Norfolk, Virginia.

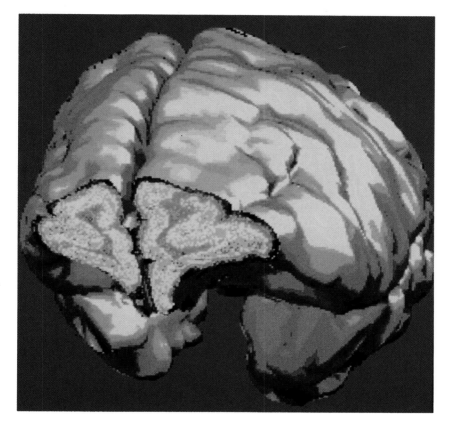

PLATE 4-3 Three-dimensional reconstruction of a monkey brain. The cortex has been rendered from histology, and the coronal section depicts glucose utilization derived from autoradiography. Image courtesy of Arthur W. Toga, Laboratory of Neuro Imaging, University of California, Los Angeles, School of Medicine.

consideration of methods to ensure confidentiality. Throughout its activities, the committee heard strong arguments against any imposed policy of data sharing. Rather, identification of the risks and disincentives to sharing should be a priority, followed by formulation of policies to provide meaningful incentives and protections for investigators who share their data. Finally, formal attention should be paid throughout the development and use of computerized resources to the ethical issues involved in data sharing, including those pertaining to the privacy of human research subjects.

Task forces and other participants explicitly identified the risks they perceived from data sharing and possible strategies for lessening those risks. First, methods must be developed to ensure that proper credit is assigned to those who contribute data for sharing—especially if the sharing is with a group that extends beyond formal collaborators. The responsibilities of the investigator who shares the data, as well as those who use the data, need to be defined. Mechanisms to protect all involved parties require careful reflection and measured policy formulation. For example, journals devoted to gene mapping and protein and gene sequencing are beginning to require that investigators deposit their raw data as a condition of publication. Participants suggested that a close examination of the benefits and difficulties attaching to these journal practices would be helpful to the neuroscience field. Another suggestion was to encourage university tenure committees in their decision-making processes to consider certain types of data sharing, particularly sharing of peer-reviewed data, as comparable to journal publication and teaching competence. It was clear from the discussions that neuroscientists, and much of the biomedical science community, are only beginning to grapple with the issues inherent in data sharing. Given this context, continued analysis and discussion are likely.

Another area of concern to participants was how to ensure that computerized resources would be accessible to more than just a few well-funded laboratories. The technological capabilities resident in neuroscience laboratories cover a fairly broad range. Restricting access by limiting the resources' usefulness to only highly sophisticated computer systems would be highly undesirable. Participants also noted, however, that the recent trends of computers becoming more powerful and, at the same time, cheaper will continue unabated. In addition, computing style eventually diffuses within specific user communities. Therefore, although initial planning phases might concentrate on more sophisticated hardware, it is likely that such computers would be generally available at lower cost only a few years down the line. Nevertheless, many participants saw the development of mechanisms to increase access across a range of technological capabilities as an important goal.

There is understandable resistance to the integration of technology into the way people work. One senior administrator, who had seen the development of computerized molecular modeling, expressed surprise about how long it took investigators to embrace the technology and begin to benefit from it (see also National Academy of Sciences, 1989). Throughout the committee's activities, awareness of this kind of resistance brought repeated cautions that it would be unreasonable to expect everyone to view the establishment of computerized resources for neuroscience with the same enthusiasm. To deal with this reality, most participants endorsed continued discussion and communication within the neuroscience community. Some even suggested that professional societies (e.g., the Society for Neuroscience) might play a role in fostering communication about these issues.

A final sociological issue raised by the committee's activities relates to changes in the work force that result from greater use of technology. It is becoming more and more common for one person in a laboratory to be the "computer expert." This person is called on to solve software problems and make the laboratory's computers work effectively to support the group's research. Ten years ago, these people were often undergraduate students, many of whom were not planning to pursue a biomedical science career. Increasingly, they are individuals who are trained in science but who also have experience and interest in the technology that supports that science, thus earning the title "scientist-programmers" (Anderson, 1989). As valuable as such people are, their career possibilities are relatively constrained. Jobs, promotions, and tenure traditionally are based on publication of research results, not the development of useful technologies to conduct research. A complementary dilemma faces computer scientists who are interested in biomedical science applications but find it difficult to publish such work in the computer science literature. Many participants stressed the value of scientist-programmers to the work of their laboratories and voiced the hope that reward structures could be improved for this new segment of the neuroscience work force.

The sociological implications of the increasing role of computer and information technology in research touch many who work in the neuroscience field (Denning, 1987), and consideration of these issues should be an integral part of planning for the future. A common theme among the topics covered in this section—sociological issues, the needed technical applications, and the development and acceptance of standard data formats—is the absence of experience on which beneficial policies can be founded. Mechanisms to gain such experience constituted a major topic of discussion for the task forces.

Strategies for Building a Base of Experience

Pilot projects are good starting points

Although uniformly supportive of the long-range goal to integrate computer and information technology into neuroscience research, all four task forces strongly recommended the establishment of pilot projects, so that a badly needed base of experience could be built. These views led to the concept of a two-phase effort. The specific kinds of pilot projects that were suggested differed from one group to another, but through communication among the task forces, the suggestions coalesced into a unified concept for the committee's consideration. Rather than separate entities, pilot projects should represent a coordinated "family" of efforts with certain goals in common. Motivating the suggestion of pilot projects was the belief that such an approach would allow "in-house" development, controlled by the eventual users of the tools and resources being examined. The importance of this kind of development was stressed by several task force members with backgrounds in database design and administration, as well as by the group that considered the Defense Mapping Agency's experience in developing computerized tools (Downs et al., 1990).

A consensus emerged that groups of investigators should constitute this pilot project program. Each of the groups would involve neuroscientists working on a specific topic, some or all of whom would be geographically separated. Task force members with experience developing databases emphasized the importance of a single, clear, unifying concept behind each group; they recommended that each group be organized around neuroscience topic areas but include clear technological goals and objectives. Most important, organization around neuroscience topics would ensure that the building of the experience base proceeded in concert with continued research and discovery about the brain and its functions.

The suggested goals of such a program were generated from discussions of research and technical needs, challenges, and opportunities, which were described in the first two sections of this chapter. Although each pilot project would not necessarily address each issue, the overall goals of the program as a whole would be the following:

• Develop digital data collection and storage methods for data at multiple levels of the neural hierarchy.

• Identify the kinds of data, level of resolution, and experimental information necessary to facilitate new insights and stimulate research.

• Examine and evaluate the various capabilities (e.g., browsing, graphic interfaces) that can increase use of the resources and enhance access to meaningful information.

• Develop a variety of databases, ranging from formal, consensus databases to informal databases for research collaboration.

• Develop and experiment with different software for translation across different computing environments, for user interfaces, for network transmission of images, for data searching, and for image generation and comparison.

• Begin to develop standard data formats, nomenclature, and data collection schemes, and to evaluate the evolution of these standards.

• Gain experience in data sharing and communication through electronic means, including networks and transportable media.

• Communicate with others in the program to share and evaluate experiences and technological developments.

The task forces considered a number of factors in relation to the neuroscience topic areas that might be chosen for the pilot project program. One was the differences among subspecialties of neuroscience in their computer "readiness"—that is, the degree to which the data in a specific field are already in digital form. For example, most of the data from human imaging studies are in digital form; a pilot group working in that area could focus its work on the goals of standards development or data sharing. In contrast, a group whose data are largely in photographic or other nondigital forms might concentrate on developing digital data collection mechanisms.

Different neuroscience subspecialties can also be separated by the "horizontal" versus "vertical" range over which they extend in the neural hierarchy. Those involved in mapping the locations of different neurotransmitters or receptors might confine the majority of their research questions horizontally to the cellular or systems levels of the hierarchy. In contrast, researchers interested in pain, sleep, or substance abuse are often interested in information that extends vertically to almost every level of the hierarchy. Because such groups may well have different data collection and management needs, including a range of neuroscience subspecialties in the pilot projects would be advantageous.

In addition to groups that vary in readiness and research focus, task force members also suggested the inclusion of groups with different kinds of computer expertise. First, individuals with programming and computer graphics expertise are needed. (Some of these experts might be scientist-programmers; others might be computer experts who lack a strong working knowledge of biology.) Second, the expertise of information technology and networking personnel should be tapped. Finally, database specialists should be involved. Again, each program group would not necessarily include all of these experts— choices would be based on the group's defined goals. The task forces recognized that the inclusion of computer and information science experts presented difficulties in that such arrangements are not typical of the personnel structure in most federally funded biomedical research projects. To offset these difficulties, task force members suggested that sources of technical expertise, such as the National Center for Biotechnology Information, university computer science departments, or supercomputer research centers, be explored to ensure on-site availability of computer science expertise.

Finally, some task force members felt it was important to include neuroscientists with various degrees of computer experience. Neuroscientists with very little experience can provide insights about the usefulness of prototype user interfaces and data organization schemes, as well as the feasibility of standards protocols and methods for converting data to digital forms. Further, communication among neuroscientists with such varied experience will ensure an understanding of the needs of the larger neuroscience community.

In summary, the task forces made specific suggestions regarding the critical need to begin to build a base of experience in the incorporation of computer and information technologies into neuroscience research. In addition, they made recommendations on the composition of pilot project groups and the goals for the overall program. To coordinate these groups and provide a focus for applying the experience they gain to the long-range goal, the task forces also recommended to the committee that a coordinating structure be established.

Coordination, oversight, and evaluation will be needed

A key area of consensus among the task forces was that pilot projects required coordination and that oversight and evaluation mechanisms were crucial to the eventual implementation of a complex of computerized resources for neuroscience (see also National Academy of Sciences, 1989). The experiences of the task force members involved with development of the genome databases underscored this need: each of the genome databases had developed independently, and interlinking these disparate systems was proving to be troublesome (Smith, 1990). On the other hand, an excess of central oversight and planning can isolate users from the development process, as occurred in the modernization efforts of the Defense Mapping Agency (Downs et al., 1990). Therefore, task force members considered it essential to establish a balance.

The structures suggested for coordination of the pilot projects were varied. Two of the task forces envisioned a multidisciplinary advisory board or committee that would be responsible for coordinating the pilot project activities and, possibly, for quality or editorial control of the contents of the database. Another task force assigned the responsibility for coordination to a host institution or core facility for each project. This host institution would document and evaluate the communication and collaboration achieved through the pilot project and evaluate standard data formats and software tools. In this scheme, the final evaluation in advance of implementing the long-range goal of a national effort would be conducted by a board composed of neuroscientists and computer scientists. Finally, the fourth task force suggested that regular meetings among the different pilot projects be held to validate data, assess needs and progress, and coordinate the exchange of software, protocols, and operational methods. In addition to these meetings, the task forces suggested that a nonprofit organization, similar to the Human Genome Organization (HUGO), be established. This organization would be responsible for long-range planning and coordination among various federal funding agencies.

The task forces did not enumerate the responsibilities appropriate to these various oversight structures. Nevertheless, they made numerous suggestions about what tasks eventually could be assigned to such boards or organizations. For example, a consensus brain database requires editors to ensure the quality and accuracy of the information it contains. In addition, the efficient use of large databases normally requires some training. Therefore, a service and educational component was recommended. Another suggestion was the establishment of boards for reviewing publications and data submitted to a comprehensive brain database.

By the close of the committee's activities, there was a strong consensus that the long-range goal of building a complex of computerized resources for neuroscience was technically feasible and that the realization of this goal would greatly enhance neuroscience research. The necessity of building a base of experience from which to realize this goal was reinforced throughout the meetings and open hearings. Key aspects of this base of experience should include the involvement of neuroscientists with computer and information scientists in pilot projects, the coordination and oversight of individual pilot projects, and careful attention to the sociological and ethical issues inherent in the use of computerized resources for science.

Funding the effort is an important issue

The committee's activities took place against the backdrop of an exceptionally difficult year in biomedical research funding. It was a year in which emergency meetings were called to assess the effects of the funding crisis on the future of biomedical science in the United States, and in which many issues of *Science* or *The Scientist* contained an article about decreasing award rates for grants or the disincentives to entering science as a career (Bloom and Randolph, 1990; Culliton, 1990; National Academy of Sciences and Institute of Medicine, 1990). Understandably, this climate left its mark on the opinions of the participants in each of the consultative activities.

Nearly all participants argued that, if the establishment of a complex of electronic and digital resources for neuroscience were important enough to undertake, appropriation of additional funds for its establishment would be necessary and justified. Most participants and respondents were enthusiastic about the potential benefits to be gained from greater integration of computerized resources in neuroscience and considered the additional investment to be justified. As might be expected, the majority of those expressing this view were neuroscientists with extensive experience in using computers for their research. Yet the task force groups and open hearings included neuroscientists with a range of computer experience. As the various meetings progressed, most neuroscientists who had moderate to minimum computer experience (and were often initially skeptical about the value of computerized resources) became excited about the advantage such tools might offer for their research. Nevertheless, despite this general enthusiasm, a few participants and respondents were opposed to the initiatives being considered—for two main reasons. First, they did not see enough benefit to justify the expenditure of funds. Second, they were concerned that the initiative might cause scarce funds to be sequestered and funneled to a small group of senior scientists. Committee members carefully considered all of these views as they developed their recommendations.

References

Anderson, G. C. 1989. New initiatives aim to emancipate "scientist-programmers." The Scientist (Sept. 18):23.

Bloom, F. E., and M. A. Randolph, eds. 1990. Funding Health Sciences Research: A Strategy to Restore Balance. Washington, D.C.: National Academy Press.

Culliton, B. J. 1990. Biomedical funding: The eternal crisis. Science 250:1652-1653.

Denning, P. J. 1987. The science of computing: A new paradigm for science. American Scientist 75:572-573.

Downs, A., B. Waxman, and C. Pechura. 1990. Technological Implications of Cartography and Remote Sensing for a National Neural Circuitry Database. Background paper prepared for the Committee on a Neural Circuitry Database, Institute of Medicine.

Fienberg, S. E., M. E. Martin, and M. L. Straf, eds. 1985. Sharing Research Data. Washington, D.C.: National Academy Press.

National Academy of Sciences. 1989. Information Technology and the Conduct of Research. Washington, D.C.: National Academy Press.

National Academy of Sciences and Institute of Medicine. 1990. Forum on Supporting Biomedical Research: Near-Term Problems and Options for Action. Summary of meeting held June 27, 1990. Washington, D.C.: National Academy Press.

Schatz, B. R. 1991. Building an Electronic Scientific Community. Pp. 739-748 in Proceedings of the 24th Annual Hawaii International Conference on Systems Sciences, IEEE Computer Society, vol. 3.

Science. 1990. What's on your mind? Check BrainMap (Briefings). Vol. 250:1203.

Smith, T. F. 1990. The history of the genetic sequence databases. Genomics 6:701-707.

Vela, C. 1990. Overview of U. S. Genome and Selected Scientific Databases. Background paper prepared for Committee on a National Neural Circuitry Database, Institute of Medicine.

Note

1. This preliminary survey was conducted by Elizabeth Meyer and Constance Pechura. For a description of the methods used, contact the Institute of Medicine, Division of Health Sciences Policy.

6
The Brain Mapping Initiative: Committee Conclusions and Recommendations

An environment of opportunity now exists to enhance neuroscience by a more global incorporation of computer and information technologies into the research enterprise. Yet it is also apparent from the experiences of other scientific disciplines, including the gene mapping community, that to ensure the greatest benefit, these technologies must be incorporated with care and with a clear vision of the intended goal. When such efforts are successfully realized, the benefit can be a great increase in our understanding of normal and pathological processes in biology. As in all biomedical research, increased knowledge and understanding lead to improvements in human health.

The Long-Range Goal

Neuroscience is immensely diverse in its methodology and levels of inquiry. To achieve true understanding, this diverse information must be coordinated into a meaningful picture. The burden of this coordination rests on individual neuroscientists, who necessarily spend the majority of their time investigating the many highly specific processes of the brain. Placing those detailed, specific data into the larger context of the multiple levels of brain organization and of all other relevant information is almost impossible—for several reasons. Neuroscience, like many other scientific fields, is divided into a range of specialties. The diversity of research methods generated by such specialization makes it unlikely that any one individual can achieve sufficient expertise in every method to allow for a learned interpretation of every reported finding in neuroscience. More important, the mass of detailed information being generated at every level of neural organization is impossible to grasp with conventional means. The investigator seeking information at even a single hierarchical level or in regard to a specific neurobiological mechanism is often daunted by how widely scattered that information may be throughout scores of different journals, review papers, symposia summaries, and books.

Computer and information sciences have made impressive advances in the past decade. The development of database technology has given all fields of science new ways of organizing and retrieving data, and research into even more sophisticated database designs is beginning to bear fruit. Emerging object-oriented database technology, for example, will permit improved manipulation and exchange of electronic images, it is hoped, by the end of this decade. Such an advance is of particular importance to neuroscience, characterized by many as a "visual science." Graphic imaging is another area of computer science that has grown rapidly to a high level of sophistication. Generation of two- and three-dimensional graphic images is becoming fast and simple, and the ability to interact with such images has endowed researchers with a high degree of flexibility in the use of these images. The combination of high-quality graphics capabilities and powerful data collection and analysis workstations promises to be an unprecedented resource for neuroscientists. It is already the case that substantial amounts of neuroscience data are collected and analyzed using a variety of computers and workstations, which run many different software programs and employ a wealth of utilities and tools. Further, the infrastructure is now under construction to link these and other, more highly developed computerized research environments through high-speed computer networks capable of transmitting text and image data in reasonable time frames.

The capabilities afforded by the recent advances in computer science now provide the opportunity to put into context the explosion of information on the brain, its circuitry, and its functions. Therefore,

the committee recommends that the Brain Mapping Initiative be established with the long-term objective of developing three-dimensional computerized maps and models of the structure, functions, connectivity, pharmacology, and molecular biology of human, rat, and monkey brains[1] across developmental stages and reflecting both normal and disease states.

The committee envisions this objective to be accomplished in two phases, beginning with phase 1 pilot projects, which will provide an experience base for the fulfillment of phase 2.

The maps and models noted above would constitute a Brain Mapping Initiative, but the committee's vision has a broader scope: not a single-entity database but a complex of interrelated, integrated databases accessible from individual laboratories. This resource would also incorporate additional tools and utilities that would allow users to interact with the data to form new associations, achieve nonstandard structural views, or otherwise change the data presentation parameters to test new hypotheses or obtain replication of specific experimental data in other systems, regions, states, or species. The committee recognizes the enormity of such an undertaking and that its successful implementation will require a transformation in the way information is acquired, communicated, and analyzed by neuroscientists.

The committee views this endeavor as a long-term project to be accomplished in two phases. Phase 1 would comprise the organized initiation of seed or pilot projects with the overall goal of gaining experience in the incorporation of the required technologies and applying that experience to the long-range planning of phase 2. In addition, pilot projects would bring focus and utility to information technology research in areas useful to neuroscience research. Phase 2 would be the construction of a complete family of maps and models—all the elements necessary to provide a complex of electronic resources to enhance neuroscience research.

Despite the broad scope and difficulty of such an effort, a number of reasons argue for initiating the project at this time. Aspects of the technological applications are, in fact, already being developed in a number of scattered prototype projects in individual neuroscience laboratories. These include prototype databases and three-dimensional reconstructions of brain structures and cells. Exchange of digital data files and data format standards is also evolving among certain neuroscientists from various subspecialties. To ensure the coordinated establishment of an integrated group of resources useful to the entire neuroscience community, however, the committee believes it is critical to plan the implementation fully and with great care. This planning should be based on experience with, for example, the use and development of standard data formats, methods of handling different kinds of data, methods of oversight and evaluation, and approaches to quality control and data security. In addition, this planning and the initial implementation steps should be managed and coordinated from the outset in a manner that facilitates cross-fertilization of ideas and openness to emerging technologies. Such coordination will further ensure the greatest general benefit and efficient use of fiscal resources through planned integration of a variety of databases and other digital resources.

Phase 1: Implementation

Phase 1 projects will be the first step in approaching the challenge

To achieve the long-range goals noted above, the committee formulated a number of other recommendations, the first of which relates to the initiation of phase 1.

> **The committee recommends the establishment of pilot projects or consortia. These projects should be peer-reviewed by neuroscientists and computer scientists; they should also be investigator initiated, involve geographically dispersed laboratories, and include neuroscientists with varied levels of computer experience. The projects should develop common formats for the exchange of data and focus on different types of computer data representations (geometric, structural, image, and free text). Selection of projects should be on the basis of research quality and value to the evolution of a complex of computerized resources for mapping the brain.**

The phase 1 projects are intended to form a base of experience and provide the necessary infrastructure for the successful development of phase 2 of the Brain Mapping Initiative—a comprehensive brain mapping effort. Each pilot project would be a consortium of several (three to six) research groups with the primary goals of mapping brain anatomy, chemistry, and functions and forging the pathways for the integration of computer and information technology into the overall neuroscience research effort. Consortia could be organized among geographically distinct institutions or as centers housed within a single institution. If the centers approach were to be adopted, special attention should be given to involving investigators from geographically distant institutions as users of the resources being developed. Although the phase 1 projects should be individually organized around specific research interests, as a whole they should represent the diversity of neuroscience questions. (That is, the organization should include both basic and clinical neuroscientific groups.) In addition, research topics should reflect the vertical hierarchy of the brain, from behavior to cells or molecules, as well as the horizontal range of inquiry, from physiological to anatomical to chemical approaches. Finally, close collaboration with computer scientists will also be necessary. Beyond these general goals, many specific issues should be addressed by the phase 1 projects, including kinds of databases, the scope of the data to be included, sociological issues, and architectural and technical requirements. These issues were discussed during task force meetings and open hearings and are summarized in Chapter 5.

The kinds of **databases** to be explored will vary because of the broad range of information that is useful to working scientists. For example, published reports from journals are a primary source of scientific data, but other, informal interactions, including scientific meetings and individual discussions, often provide scientists with deeper understanding. The databases developed for the neuroscience field should attempt to include both kinds of information. Phase 1 projects could investigate the usefulness of the following kinds of databases: reference databases, data banks, informal databases, international registries and directories, research collaboration databases, and specialty databases (see Chapter 5). Each of these database forms needs to be thoroughly investigated by phase 1 projects; however, certain resources should be implemented immediately.

> **The committee recognizes that neuroscience efforts proceed internationally and recommends that an international registry of neuroscience databases and contacts be established so that appropriate linkages can be created in the future.**

Such a registry, which should be available through computer networks, would help to identify what resources are currently available and also provide a mechanism by which efforts could be coordinated. Further, it would enable current investigators to develop interaction with others with whom data collection strategies, design problems and solutions, and other related issues could be discussed. It is expected that such a registry would initially contain very few groups or databases but that it would grow as the phase 1 projects proceeded.

> **The committee recommends the establishment of an archive of public domain software, accessible through computer networks.**

The committee expects that phase 1 projects will have special needs for novel software. Public domain software is available at little or no cost to anyone who wants to use it, and these programs should be explored. In addition, such an archive would encourage the formation of neuroscience "news groups," or groups of users with similar interests, who could communicate by computer bulletin boards or electronic mail.

The **scope of the data** to be included in phase 1 projects must be broad to be genuinely useful to neuroscience research, both immediately and eventually for phase 2. Although some kinds of data have universal applicability to all branches of neuroscience, other kinds are necessary only for specialized groups of investigators. In addition, the range of data covered should include normal and pathological states; it should also reflect changes that occur during development and aging. In many respects, the kinds of data to be included are relatively easy to define. The incorporation of diverse types into a unified whole, however, will present a sizable challenge to phase 1 investigators and managers.

There was consensus among the task forces and support from the wider neuroscience community that anatomical data were the key data element and might well serve as the "backbone" with which other data types can be associated (see Chapter 5). An analogy can be made that basic brain anatomical maps or atlases are similar to LANDSAT images. Detailed information, such as precise connections, neurochemistry, cell types, and physiological response properties, can all be mapped onto those basic images in much the same way roads and other landmarks can be mapped onto LANDSAT images (Downs et al., 1990). Moreover, the level of resolution can change in both LANDSAT and brain images: it can be adjusted up or down depending on the sensitivity of the "sensors" employed. Thus, the location of pyramidal cells in a particular cortical area could be mapped from medium-magnification light microscopic examination. From higher level magnification (light or electron microscope), the differential location of neurotransmitter substances or receptors could be mapped onto a three-dimensional reconstruction of the pyramidal cell. At yet a higher level, using sensitive electrophysiological sensors, the differential locations of ion channels could be mapped. Such maps, which are prepared now largely by hand, are important contributions to the construction of computational models of neuronal function.

As outlined in Chapter 5, **sociological issues** present some of the most vexing problems in establishing any database or implementing any large-scale initiative. Such matters are intimately joined with how people work on a daily basis, the traditions they hold, and, often more important, how they are invested personally in their work. Understandable sensitivity exists in such areas, and careful attention to these issues is necessary for those involved with the development and planning of electronic resources.

Including investigators with different levels of computer expertise in phase 1 projects will facilitate greater acceptance of computer technology by emphasizing the varied needs of the neuroscience community and opening important channels of communication. In terms of data-sharing, the committee assigns no value judgment to either end of the continuum of possible actions; that a continuum exists, however, must be recognized and dealt with. The priority that phase 1 projects place on establishing collaborative groups will dictate that attention be paid to data-sharing mechanisms. As part of this effort, phase 1 projects should explore methods to ensure that preliminary data are clearly labeled and that proper credit will be given to those who contribute data for sharing. The committee also encourages examination of the effects of policies already in place—those developed by the journals devoted to gene mapping and protein and gene sequencing—that require data deposit as a condition of publication. In addition, the committee supports the concept that university tenure committees should begin to consider which kinds of data sharing should be viewed as evidence of professional competence, comparable to journal publication and teaching evaluations.

If electronic resources are to be accepted and utilized, scientists must trust the accuracy of the information contained within the resource. Therefore, phase 1 projects must begin to find ways to ensure such accuracy, especially of information included in reference databases, data banks, and registries. Mechanisms are needed to ensure the appropriate use of different levels of data and to permit the deletion of information that becomes obsolete. Such mechanisms may include management of the database by an editor (or group of editors) who is an expert in the field and whose function would be analogous to that of a journal editor.

Another important sociological issue facing phase 1 projects is the acceptance of standards for data representation, data entry, nomenclature, and methods of data annotation. Currently accepted methods of representing data lack the level of precision required for coordinated computer resources. The committee thus agrees with the views of task force and other study participants that such standards are needed but that they should evolve from experience and should be based on the needs of users, rather than imposed from some outside source.

In terms of the proposed complex's **technical and architectural requirements**, definition and specification are impossible in the absence of a concerted, hands-on effort to construct a usable computer resource. The committee received valuable advice from its members, from task force participants, and from other experts with experience in these kinds of efforts (see Chapter 5), and this advice is encompassed in a general framework in four areas that should be explored by phase 1 investigators. Database management technology is the first: in database planning, phase 1 investigators are encouraged to seek input from such resources as the National Center for Biotechnology Information at the National Library of Medicine and from national supercomputing centers, including the National Center for Super-computing Applications and the Ohio and Pittsburgh Supercomputing Centers. Particularly desirable is the involvement of established, successful university programs in biomedical computing research.

Computer networks are the second technical requirement area to be considered. The future of national and international computer networks is particularly promising for the development of a brain mapping effort. The committee strongly endorses international expansion of Internet, implementation of the proposed National Research and Education Network, and the upgrades planned for existing wide area network infrastructures, such as NSFNET. Phase 1 projects should keep abreast of the developments in network capabilities and remain aware of the policies that underlie concomitant upgrades of university-controlled local area networks.

Compatibility of computer hardware and operating systems is the third area for consideration in the architectural and technical requirements for a brain mapping effort. It will be important to identify the operating systems that neuroscientists use and to develop software that runs on various kinds of systems. Another approach to compatibility is the design of data interchange formats that allow for translation from one software program to another. These and other approaches should be explored; however, care should be taken not to limit compatibility by limiting access. A balance should be struck between advanced access mechanisms, such as high-speed networks, and more traditional mechanisms, such as telephone-based connections among personal computers. In addition, different kinds of data storage options should be explored.

Finally, there are technical issues relating to the development of standards, as well as the sociological issues mentioned in the previous section. The identification of effective standards should be an early priority for phase 1 projects because the initial design of databases and communication protocols must take such standards into consideration. In this area, the committee encourages interaction between phase 1 investigators and the Internet Activities Board's Engineering Task Force, which conducts specific development projects for network data transmission. The committee also suggests cooperation with the National Information Standards Organization (NISO), which is responsible for the development of standards for library applications.

Phase 1 projects should be centrally organized

For phase 1 projects to provide the proper basis for the development of a coordinated brain mapping effort, communication among the consortia and some type of central oversight are needed.

The committee recommends that an administrative structure be established to coordinate phase 1 activities. This Brain Map Advisory Panel (BMAP) should be composed of neuroscientists and computer and information scientists, with additional input from funding agency administrators. The panel would be responsible for the overall direction, evaluation, and coordination of consortia and for the development of necessary policies relating to establishment of a brain mapping effort. The committee also recommends that the Advisory Panel be responsible for consideration and development of editorial functions and policies relating to the ethical and sociological issues that will arise, including, but not limited to, correctness of information and quality control, intellectual property rights, rights to privacy, and freedom of information.

The panel could also coordinate action by funding agencies and other, related scientific initiatives. Finally, the panel would undertake the long-range planning of phase 2.

As described earlier, the issues confronting the phase 1 projects are many and diverse, ranging from sociological to highly technical areas. Each of the consortia will need the kind of central clearinghouse for information that the proposed panel can provide. For example, the panel can examine various approaches to database design and weigh the outcomes against the scientific needs of both specialized groups and the neuroscience community as a whole. Of particular value to the coordinating function of the BMAP would be to establish contacts with other groups, including the astrophysics, earth mapping, and global change research communities, to share information and discuss common issues. An additional resource might be the Telescience Testbed Program of the National Aeronautics and Space Administration.

The panel can also collate measures of the actual use of developing resources and of successful incentives for data sharing from among the various consortia to obtain a clear picture of what works and what does not. In addition, the panel could gather information from the consortia about emerging trends in the computer industry that might affect the development of phase 2, suggest more efficient data-handling methods, or facilitate more effective communication protocols.

Mechanisms for integrating the developing technologies into the work practices of neuroscientists will be another area of the panel's concern. Providing quality service, education, and training is essential for the sharing and effective use of research data. The panel's role in phase 1 should be to develop an infrastructure to provide these components. Appropriate services would include reliable access, distribution of data through a variety of means, and documentation of database contents. In addition, consulting support for local problems will be needed. Phase 2 efforts will also require several kinds of training at diverse sites and the development of training materials. Inclusion of panels and demonstrations at relevant scientific meetings should be explored as options. The construction of a dynamic infrastructure will promote strong interaction among development, service, and educational activities that will significantly increase the usefulness of the resource.

The oversight provided by the panel should not occur in a completely "top-down" manner because such an approach could isolate the consortia from each other and slow the transfer of important findings and developments. Mechanisms should be found for organized cross-communication among the consortia and the panel. One way to accomplish this communication would be to include representatives from each consortium on the panel. Another mechanism that deserves serious consideration is to hold regular meetings of consortia investigators. Such an approach has been successful for certain genome databases. For example, the principal investigators from each consortium could meet semiannually or quarterly to present their work and identify the advances made and the barriers encountered. The meetings thus would provide the opportunity to validate data, assess needs and progress, and coordinate the exchange of software, protocols, and operational methods. They might also be used as a vehicle to obtain input from experts in neuroscience, computer science, or industry who are not involved in the phase 1 projects or on the panel but who have special skills that can be brought to bear on particular problems and issues. The panel could also participate in these meetings to offer input, receive requests for needed action, and provide a record of the proceedings.

Another responsibility of the panel would be to coordinate the establishment of the international registry of neuroscience databases and contacts, and the archive of public domain software that the committee has recommended be established. In addition, the coordination of phase 1 projects with other national and international efforts is extremely important. Therefore,

the committee recommends that the phase 1 and 2 projects of the Brain Mapping Initiative maintain a close relationship with the gene mapping and sequencing community and

the Human Genome Project, and with other scientific computing efforts, including network initiatives such as NSFNET and the proposed National Research and Education Network. As part of these efforts, the committee further recommends that linkages be established with protein sequence and genome databases to enhance access to information about brain-specific genes.

Phase 1 projects will require additional funding

Special challenges related to funding confront the implementation of the phase 1 projects. The first is to determine a basic funding approach. There are three ways in which federal dollars are provided for biomedical research. One is by a contract mechanism in which a government agency funds projects that it proposes, which are completed by an outside investigator according to a contract written by the government agency. The government agencies then oversee and supervise such projects. Contract mechanisms are often used by the Department of Defense to fund research, but they represent a much smaller portion of the funding provided by NIH and ADAMHA for biomedical research (ADAMHA, 1988; National Institutes of Health, 1989). The other mechanism, which is more typical of ADAMHA, NIH, and NSF funding, is that of grants to investigators or groups of investigators for research projects that are proposed, accomplished, and supervised by the investigators themselves (investigator-initiated). The third funding mechanism, cooperative agreements involving researchers and their universities, is currently used by the NSF for some projects and functions like a combination grant/contract. The committee received a great deal of input about the relative merits of these mechanisms, especially regarding grants versus contracts. Generally, it favors the use of grant mechanisms and cooperative agreements for funding the proposed initiative. This judgment is based on the committee's belief that the development of usable resources should be intricately combined with the research itself, and this dual task can best be done by scientists actively involved in the research. The limited use of contracts, however, may confer advantages during some aspects of phase 1 activities. Therefore,

the committee recommends that federal funding agencies develop requests for applications and/or cooperative agreements to support the formation of consortia and the activities of the Brain Map Advisory Panel. Limited use of contract mechanisms should also be considered when appropriate to the overall goals of the initiative.

The second challenge is the fact that the proposed phase 1 organization is not typical of the current administrative or funding structures employed by the federal agencies responsible for the biomedical sciences. The typical structure of NIH and ADAMHA funding is that individual institutes provide funding for individual grants (R01s) or program project grants (P01s) for specific research projects related to the institute's overall research program goals. Review of such grants on the basis of scientific merit is accomplished either through the NIH Division of Research Grants' study sections or through an individual institute's scientific review groups.

The proposed oversight panel and consortia, each consisting of groups of investigators (similar to program project groups), constitute a structure the committee considers essential to the success of the Brain Mapping Initiative. Such a structure, however, will require flexibility in the typical biomedical funding mechanisms noted above and cooperation among different agencies. The committee is not recommending a reorganization of the federal biomedical research complex; nevertheless, it sees a critical need for greater communication and cooperation among the components of the complex. Further, this communication and cooperation might be extended to include agencies outside the Public Health Service, such as the Departments of Defense and Energy, as well as private agencies, foundations, and universities that provide resources for biomedical science. To this end,

> **the committee recommends that phases 1 and 2 of the Brain Mapping Initiative be international in scope and that they be funded by multiple sources in a coordinated fashion. The structure for administering the funding should ensure program stability and effectiveness. Possible funding structures include the identification of a lead agency or institute, or the establishment of formal administrative structures among two or more agencies.**

The committee is also sensitive to the current fiscal restraints on the entire U.S. biomedical research effort (National Academy of Sciences and Institute of Medicine, 1990; Lederman, 1991). Given this reality, there is understandable concern among scientists that large initiatives pose a threat to the survival or health of individual investigator-based research. In the case of the Brain Mapping Initiative, these fears are unfounded. The project proposed here would constitute a very small part of the entire neuroscience research effort. Moreover, the history of neuroscience abounds with examples of how technological advances have provided the tools with which major discoveries have been made, discoveries that have led directly to significant reductions in human suffering. Incorporation of computer science and information technology, to their full potential, into neuroscience research represents a technological advance that will be analogous to, and may even rival, the development of the oscilloscope and the electron microscope. It is important to reiterate that these proposals are aimed toward coordinating what would be widely separated activities into a unified effort. Only an effort of this kind can provide the kind of coordination and careful planning for the future that uses scarce resources efficiently and effectively and ensures greater use of the emerging technology by the neuroscience community as a whole. Therefore,

> **the committee concludes that the expected benefits of the proposed Brain Mapping Initiative justify the investment of necessary resources and recommends the appropriation of additional funding to support the establishment of phase 1 projects.**

Phase 1 projects will require a certain amount of time and support

Five years is the minimum time that should be allowed for phase 1 projects to reach the level of expertise and technological development necessary to initiate phase 2. Further, as phase 2 is initiated, the phase 1 projects should be kept in place—for a period of time to be determined by the Advisory Panel—and, possibly, phased out gradually as phase 2 begins or simply incorporated into the larger initiative.

The budget for phase 1 can be estimated at $10 million per year, with an expected duration of five years. This amount is based on establishing five consortia groups, each with a $2 million-per-year funding level. The $2 million would be distributed among consortia participants; thus, individual funding levels could range from $200,000 to $400,000 annually. This funding would be used to cover the costs of investigator research support, computer systems, software and software development, establishment of necessary local area networks, and travel for consortia participants. The Advisory Panel would also require support from these funds to cover travel and administrative costs.

Phase 2: Long-Term Integration and Its Potential Benefits

The brain presents some of the most fascinating, complex questions in biological science. Neuroscience has amassed a substantial body of knowledge about the structures of the brain and their specific functions, but in many ways this mass of knowledge is only a beginning. It is now time to fit the millions of pieces of the puzzle into place and bring neuroscience to a point at which it can begin to alter the course of many diseases and disabilities. The proposed Brain Mapping Initiative will allow investigators studying the brain to view data in new ways, to share data with each other, and to access needed data from any of the neuroscience subspecialties. So enabled, neuroscientists will map the brain and its functions to a degree only faintly imaginable even 20 years ago. The brain map that is thus generated can be reasonably expected to contribute greatly to the improvement of human health and the alleviation of some of the most mysterious and intractable of human diseases.

Our society faces an already large and still growing burden from diseases that affect the brain. Many of these diseases are multifactorial, making them difficult to understand and difficult to treat. For example, addiction to cocaine and other drugs has reached epidemic proportions (Gerstein and Harwood, 1990). Understanding the receptor systems of the brain that mediate these drugs' effects and the brain regions that are affected is critical to achieve the kind of useful treatments that have eluded us for years. But the problem becomes exceedingly more difficult if the secondary effects of drug abuse are considered. A 1988 national household survey conducted by the Research Triangle Institute and the National Institute on Drug Abuse indicated that about 9.3 million women in high-fertility age brackets (15–35 years) had used an illicit drug at least once in the year previous to the survey. With the overall expected birth rate for a group in this age bracket taken into account, these figures suggest a probable range of 350,000 to 625,000 annual fetal exposures to one or more episodes of maternal drug consumption (Gerstein and Harwood, 1990; U.S. General Accounting Office, 1990). Not only are many of these babies born addicted to drugs, but the development of their brains has been altered, leading to attention deficits and learning disabilities, among other problems. We need desperately to understand and treat drug addiction, but we also need to understand and treat or prevent the developmental deficits it causes. The pressure to accomplish these goals is increasing rapidly. In another five years, the drug-damaged children born this year will be entering the school systems of many large cities in the United States. These schools will also be dealing with other children who have been neurologically damaged—as a result of malnutrition, lead poisoning, lack of adequate maternal prenatal care, and untreated childhood diseases (Institute of Medicine, 1989). The resulting toll on our precious human resources is obvious.

Every year, half a million children and adults experience brain and spinal cord injuries (National Advisory Neurological and Communicative Disorders and Stroke Council, 1989). Most often, these injuries lead to paralysis and lifelong disabilities. The mass of neuroscience research conducted to date has brought us to the threshold of being able to prevent the devastating effects of these injuries, but traversing that threshold will depend on the discoveries to be made in the next decade. The same conditions apply to the treatment and prevention of Alzheimer's disease. In the previous decade, we identified some of the locations of damage caused by this disease, documented some of the biochemical processes that are associated with that damage, and tested a variety of pharmacological agents for their ability to slow the disease process. Yet here again, we merely stand at the threshold.

It is enlightening to remember that virtually every system of the body is affected by brain activity either through the central nervous system or the peripheral nerves that constitute the sensory systems and the autonomic nervous system. Thus, the study of neuroscience has the potential to contribute to the development of treatments for many diseases that are typically not considered neurological—for example, certain endocrine disorders, cardiac arrhythmias, and gastric ulcers. In addition, many systemic disease processes result in neurological problems that often have a metabolic basis but that are not completely understood. Examples of these problems include the chronic pain and nerve disorders that result from diabetes and the mental retardation caused by thyroid insufficiency.

An excellent climate of opportunity currently prevails to expand our knowledge of brain functioning during the coming decade. Seizing this opportunity, however, requires a concerted, interdisciplinary effort on the part of basic and clinical neuroscientists worldwide. It is becoming clear that the scientific enterprise in general relies increasingly on the use of sophisticated methodologies and computer technologies. This committee has considered how the full potential of computer technologies in neuroscience research can be realized. It strongly believes that realization of this potential through the establishment of the Brain Mapping Initiative is essential to ensure the greatest benefit to society from neuroscience research.

Summary of Recommendations

1. The committee recommends that the Brain Mapping Initiative be established with the long-term objective of developing three-dimensional computerized maps and models of the structure, functions, connectivity, pharmacology, and molecular biology of human, rat, and monkey brains across developmental stages and reflecting both normal and disease states. The committee envisions this objective to

be accomplished in two phases, beginning with phase 1 pilot projects, which will provide an experience base for the fulfillment of phase 2.

2. The committee recommends the establishment of pilot projects or consortia. These projects should be peer-reviewed by neuroscientists and computer scientists; they should also be investigator initiated, involve geographically dispersed laboratories, and include neuroscientists with varied levels of computer experience. The projects should develop common formats for the exchange of data and focus on dif-ferent types of computer data representations (geometric, structural, image, and free text). Selection of projects should be on the basis of research quality and value to the evolution of a complex of electronic resources for mapping the brain.

3. The committee recognizes that neuroscience efforts proceed internationally and recommends that an international registry of neuroscience databases and contacts be established so that appropriate linkages can be created in the future.

4. The committee recommends the establishment of an archive of public domain software, accessible through computer networks.

5. The committee recommends that an administrative structure be established to coordinate phase 1 activities. This Brain Map Advisory Panel (BMAP) should be composed of neuroscientists and computer and information scientists, with additional input from funding agency administrators. The panel would be responsible for the overall direction, evaluation, and coordination of consortia and for the development of necessary policies relating to establishment of a brain mapping effort. The committee also recommends that the Advisory Panel be responsible for consideration and development of editorial functions and policies relating to the ethical and sociological issues that will arise, including, but not limited to, correctness of information and quality control, intellectual property rights, rights to privacy, and freedom of information.

6. The committee recommends that the phase 1 and 2 projects of the Brain Mapping Initiative maintain a close relationship with the gene mapping and sequencing community and the Human Genome Project, and with other scientific computing efforts, including network initiatives such as NSFNET and the proposed National Research and Education Network. As part of these efforts, the committee further recommends that linkages be established with protein sequence and genome databases to enhance access to information about brain-specific genes.

7. The committee recommends that federal funding agencies develop requests for applications and/or cooperative agreements to support the formation of consortia and the activities of the Brain

Map Advisory Panel. Limited use of contract mechanisms should also be considered when appropriate to the overall goals of the initiative.

8. The committee recommends that phases 1 and 2 of the Brain Mapping Initiative be international in scope and that they be funded by multiple sources in a coordinated fashion. The structure for administering the funding should ensure program stability and effectiveness. Possible funding structures include the identification of a lead agency or institute, or the establishment of formal administrative structures among two or more agencies.

9. The committee concludes that the expected benefits of the proposed Brain Mapping Initiative justify the investment of necessary resources and recommends the appropriation of additional funding to support the establishment of phase 1 projects.

References

Alcohol, Drug Abuse, and Mental Health Administration (ADAMHA). 1988. ADAMHA Funding Mechanisms for Grants and Awards. Rockville, Md.: U.S. Department of Health and Human Services.

Downs, A., B. Waxman, and C. Pechura. 1990. Technological Implications of Cartography and Remote Sensing for a National Neural Circuitry Database. Background paper prepared for the Committee on a National Neural Circuitry Database, Institute of Medicine.

Gerstein, D. R., and H. J. Harwood, eds. 1990. Treating Drug Problems, vol. 1. Washington, D.C.: National Academy Press

Institute of Medicine. 1989. Research on Children and Adolescents with Mental, Behavioral, and Developmental Disorders: Mobilizing a National Initiative. Washington, D.C.: National Academy Press.

Lederman, L. M. 1991. Science: The End of the Frontier? Science 251(Jan. 11, insert): 1-19.

National Academy of Sciences and Institute of Medicine. 1990. Forum on Supporting Biomedical Research: Near-Term Problems and Options for Action. Summary of meeting held June 27, 1990. Washington, D.C.: National Academy Press.

National Advisory Neurological and Communicative Disorders and Stroke Council. 1989. Decade of the Brain: Answers Through Scientific Research. NIH Pub. No. 88-2957. Bethesda, Md.: U.S. Department of Health and Human Services, National Institutes of Health.

National Institutes of Health. 1989. NIH Data Book. Pub. No. 90-1261. Bethesda, Md.: U.S. Department of Health and Human Services.

U.S. General Accounting Office. 1990. Drug Exposed Infants: A Generation at Risk. Testimony before the Committee on Finance, U.S. Senate. Pub. No. GAO/T-HRD-90-46. Washington, D.C.: U.S. General Accounting Office.

Note

1. These species are intended as starting points. The committee also recognizes the need to include data from other, vertebrate and invertebrate, species.

Appendixes

A

Task Force Topics and Rosters

Task Force 1

Task Force 1 met in Washington, D.C. on January 30 and 31, 1990. The group examined the issues related to establishing a complex of automated resources for neuroscience research from the perspective of those working in neurophysiology, neuroanatomy, and other fields in which the hierarchical character of neural systems must be considered.

Gordon M. Shepherd,* Yale University School of Medicine
Vinton Cerf,* Corporation for National Research Initiatives
David G. Amaral, Salk Institute
Joseph Capowski, Eutectics Electronics
Edward G. Jones, University of California, Irvine, College of Medicine
David Lipman, National Center for Biotechnology Information
Clifford Lynch, University of California, Oakland
David A. McCormick, Yale University School of Medicine
Scooter Morris, Genentech
Clint Potter, National Center for Supercomputing Applications
Bruce Schatz, University of Arizona
Terrence J. Sejnowski, Salk Institute

---

*Member, Institute of Medicine Committee on a National Neural Circuitry Database.

Task Force 2

Task Force 2 met in Washington, D.C. on February 1 and 2, 1990. The group examined the relevant issues in relation to mapping the presence of neurotransmitters, receptors, or changes in glucose metabolism, blood flow, or ion concentration in specific regions of the brain (i.e., autoradiographic and densitometric data).

Joseph T. Coyle,* Johns Hopkins University School of Medicine
Diane C.P. Smith,* Xerox Corporation
Michael J. Kuhar, NIDA Addiction Research Center
Charles Molnar, Washington University
Virginia M. Pickel, Cornell University, School of Medicine
Arthur W. Toga, University of California, Los Angeles
Oleh Tretiak, Drexel University
Stanley J. Watson, University of Michigan School of Medicine
Turner Whitted, Numerical Design Ltd.
William Yamamoto, George Washington University Medical Center

Task Force 3

Task Force 3 met in Irvine, California, on March 5 and 6, 1990. The group examined the issues from the perspective of those involved in human brain imaging, including PET scanning, MRI visualization, CT scanning, and the combination or overlaying of these images.

Marcus E. Raichle,* Washington University School of Medicine
Jerome R. Cox,* Washington University
Karen J. Berkley,* Florida State University
Verne S. Caviness, Massachusetts General Hospital
Alan Evans, Montreal Neurological Institute
Peter Fox, Johns Hopkins University School of Medicine
David LaBerge, University of California, Irvine
Martin Reite, University of Colorado
Larry Squire, Veterans Administration Medical Center, San Diego
Chris Wood, Los Alamos National Laboratory

Task Force 4

Task Force 4 met in Irvine, California, on March 7 and 8, 1990, and examined the issues in relation to the generation of a comprehensive

---

*Member, Institute of Medicine Committee on a National Neural Circuitry Database.

brain mapping project aimed toward the storage and possible display of organized knowledge about the structure and functions of the brain.

Donald J. Woodward,* University of Texas Health Science Center
James Kajiya,* California Institute of Technology
Floyd E. Bloom, Scripps Clinic and Research Foundation
Dean Hillman, New York University Medical Center
Richard Lucier,* Johns Hopkins University School of Medicine
Bruce McCormick, Texas A & M University
George Paxinos, University of New South Wales, Australia
Larry W. Swanson,* University of Southern California
David Van Essen,* California Institute of Technology
James Winget, Silicon Graphics
Kwang-I Yu, TRW

---

*Member, Institute of Medicine Committee on a National Neural Circuitry Database.

B

Samples of
Requests for Opinions

The following request for opinions was published in the *Society for Neuroscience Newsletter, Trends in Neuroscience, Communications of the Association for Computing Machinery (ACM)*, and the *Journal of NIH Research.*

Request for Opinions
Concerning a National Neural Circuitry Database

The Institute of Medicine of the National Academy of Sciences has formed a study committee to examine the desirability, feasibility, and possible ways of establishing a National Neural Circuitry Database (NNCD). It is planned that the report of this committee, including specific recommendations, will be issued in January 1991. Under consideration is an NNCD that would contain textual and graphic information on the anatomy, physiology, chemistry, and pharmacology of rat, monkey, and human brains. The database would, through two- and three-dimensional graphic display, permit the users to rotate or slice images in order to access various types of information regarding brain structure and function. Further, such a database could allow for the electronic storage and transmission of neuroscience data; thus, the database could function as a vehicle for basic and clinical neuroscience research collaboration and data sharing.

The study committee recognizes the critical need for any eventual NNCD to be planned carefully with the highest priority assigned to the needs of the potential users in the neuroscience community. Therefore, the committee invites any interested persons to offer their opinions, suggestions and/or concerns on this matter in writing to:

Constance Pechura, Ph.D.
National Academy of Sciences
Institute of Medicine, Room 324
2101 Constitution Avenue, N.W.
Washington, D.C. 20418

Please confine your comments to no more than two, single-spaced, typewritten pages. It would be most useful if comments were received by *April 30, 1990,* but all comments received by May 31, 1990, will be considered.

The study is being conducted by the Institute of Medicine/National Academy of Sciences with funds provided by the National Institute of Mental Health, National Institute on Drug Abuse, and National Science Foundation.

The following letter was sent to the current and past presidents and councilors of the Society for Neuroscience.

December 21, 1989

Dear⎯⎯⎯⎯⎯⎯⎯⎯⎯⎯⎯ :

There have been discussions among members of the Society for Neuroscience for a number of years regarding the ever-burgeoning amount of data generated by neuroscience research and how the management of this vast knowledge base is becoming impossible for individual investigators. Such discussions often include the possibility of establishing some kind of database for neuroscience, and a few neuroscientists have begun to develop small, prototype databases for their own areas of interest. In response to these interests, the National Institute of Mental Health, National Institute on Drug Abuse, and the National Science Foundation have requested the Institute of Medicine/ National Academy of Sciences to form a study committee to examine the desirability, feasibility, and possible ways of establishing a National Neural Circuitry Database (NNCD). I agreed to chair this committee, composed of neuroscientists and computer scientists, because I believe that such a project requires the kind of careful consideration and objective assessment that an IOM study can provide. In addition, although the usefulness of an NNCD might be imagined, the actual establishment of such a resource would present a daunting challenge in terms of organization, planning, and funding. Therefore,

I would like the committee to draw from as broad a range of experience and expertise as possible. With that commitment in mind, I am inviting you, the current and past presidents and councilors of the Society for Neuroscience, to offer your thoughts, suggestions, and concerns regarding our study.

The kind of NNCD that we have been charged to assess would be intended as a resource for basic and clinical neuroscience. It would not be a simple bibliographic reference source; rather, it would contain textual and graphic information on the anatomy, physiology, chemistry, and pharmacology of rat, monkey, and human brains. It is envisioned that the database would, through two- and three-dimensional graphic displays, permit the users to rotate or slice images in order to access various types of information about brain structure and function. Further, such a database could allow for the electronic storage and transmission of neuroscience data; thus, it could function as a vehicle for research collaboration and data sharing.

Although we also intend to request opinions from neuroscientists through published solicitations and open forum meetings, I feel that your experience in the leadership of the Society can lend a special perspective to this issue. Please send your reply to the IOM study director, Dr. Constance Pechura (listed below); she will compile the responses and send copies to me. Connie will also be available by phone if you have any questions or need any additional information.

I greatly appreciate your time and thought in responding to this request.

With best regards in the New Year,

Sincerely,

Joseph B. Martin, M.D., Ph.D.
Chairman
Committee on a National
Neural Circuitry Database

C

Lists of Speakers and Demonstrators in Symposia and Open Hearings

Neuroscience Symposium and Open Hearing
National Academy of Sciences
Washington, D.C.
June 15, 1990

CARLA J. SHATZ
  Stanford University School of Medicine
  "Correlated neural activity and visual system development"
RICHARD J. ROBERTS
  Cold Spring Harbor Laboratory
  "Predictive sequence motifs in proteins"
GORDON SHEPHERD*
  Yale University School of Medicine
  Open Hearing: "Creating a national neuroscience resource"

---

*Member, Institute of Medicine Committee on a National Neural Circuitry Database.

Washington Computer Demonstrations

WARREN YOUNG
  Scripps Clinic & Research Foundation
STEVE WERTHEIM
  Harvard University
STEVE GREENBERG, WALLY WELKER
  University of Wisconsin
ARTHUR TOGA
  University of California, Los Angeles

Neuroscience Symposium and Open Hearing
University of California
San Francisco
June 26, 1990

ROBERT L. MACDONALD
  University of Michigan
  "Regulation of single channel properties
    of native and cloned $GABA_A$ receptors"
ROBERT LANGRIDGE
  University of California, San Francisco
  "Computational molecular biology"
DAVID VAN ESSEN*
  California Institute of Technology
  Open Hearing: "Creating a national neuroscience resource"

San Francisco Computer Demonstrations

WARREN YOUNG
  Scripps Clinic & Research Foundation
ARTHUR TOGA
  University of California, Los Angeles
JONATHAN NISSANOV
  Drexel University

---

*Member, Institute of Medicine Committee on a National Neural Circuitry Database.

Neuroscience Symposium and Open Hearing
Northwestern University
Chicago, Illinois
July 12, 1990

CHRISTOF KOCH
  California Institute of Technology
  "Computing optical flow in men, monkeys, and machines"
PETER L. PEARSON
  The Johns Hopkins University
  "The development and implementation of databases
     for mapping the human genome"
DONALD WOODWARD*
  University of Texas Health Science Center
  Open Hearing: "Creating a national neuroscience resource"

Chicago Computer Demonstrations

STEVE WERTHEIM
  Harvard University
ARTHUR TOGA
  University of California, Los Angeles
STEVE GREENBERG
  University of Wisconsin
JONATHAN NISSANOV
  Drexel University

---

*Member, Institute of Medicine Committee on a National Neural Circuitry Database.

Index

143